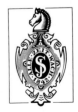

Late Reconstructions
of Injured
Ligaments of the Knee

Edited by
K.-P. Schulitz H. Krahl W. H. Stein

With Contributions by
M. E. Blazina D. H. O'Donoghue S. L. James
J. C. Kennedy A. Trillat

With 42 Figures

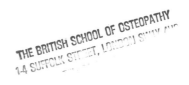
Springer-Verlag
Berlin Heidelberg New York 1978

Professor Dr. KLAUS-PETER SCHULITZ, Orthopädische Klinik und Poliklinik der Universität Düsseldorf, Moorenstr. 3, D-4000 Düsseldorf

Professor Dr. HARTMUT KRAHL and Dr. WOLFGANG HANS STEIN, Orthopädische Klinik und Poliklinik der Universität Heidelberg Schlierbacher Landstr. 200 a, D-6900 Heidelberg-Schlierbach

Contributions given at a 1977 workshop in Heidelberg at the invitation of the above mentioned editors.

ISBN 3-540-08720-6 Springer-Verlag Berlin Heidelberg New York
ISBN 0-387-08720-6 Springer-Verlag New York Heidelberg Berlin

CIP-Kurztitelaufnahme der Deutschen Bibliothek. Late reconstructions of injured ligaments of the knee / ed. by K.-P. Schulitz. With contributions by M. E. Blazina. – Berlin, Heidelberg, New York: Springer, 1978. NE: Schulitz, Klaus-Peter [Hrsg.]; Blazina, M. E. [Mitarb.]

Offsetprinting and Bookbinding: Konrad Triltsch, Graphischer Betrieb, 8700 Würzburg. 2123/3130-543210

Contents

Introduction 1

1. Surgical Anatomy of the Knee. S.L. JAMES. With 6 Figures 3
   Medial Side of the Knee 3
   Posterior Structures of the Knee 7
   Lateral Structures 9
   Cruciate Ligaments 11
   Menisci 13
   Suggested Reading 14
   Discussion 15

2. Biomechanics of the Ligaments of the Knee. J.C. KENNEDY 19
   Method of Measurement 19
   Laboratory Testing and Results 20
   Importance of Tests for Clinical Practice 21

3. Biomechanic Discussion of the Polyflex Ligament. M.E. BLAZINA.
   With 2 Figures 22
   Properties of Richards Polyflex Ligament...................... 23
   Results of Laboratory Testing 23
   Clinical Experience and Suggestions for Improvement 25
   Discussion 27

4. Classification of Knee Joint Instability Resulting From Liga-
   mentous Damage. J.C. KENNEDY 33
   Classification 33
   Discussion 34
   Description of Classification 34
       A. One-Plane Instabilities 34
       B. Rotatory Instabilities 35
       C. Combined Instabilities 36
   Discussion 37

5. Diagnosis of Different Instabilities. D.H. O'DONOGHUE. With 11
   Figures 40
   Goals of Treatment 40
   Clinical Picture 40
   Clinical Aspects of Knee Anatomy 41
   Location of Injury 43
   Method of Examination 44
   References 50

6. Assessment of Chronic Ligamentous Instability Using Arthrography,
   Arthroscopy, and Anesthesia. M.E. BLAZINA. With 1 Figure 51
   Diagnosis Using Normal Clinical Methods 52
   Diagnostic Use of Arthrography 53
   Diagnostic Use of Arthroscopy 55
   Examination Under Anesthesia 56
   Discussion 57

7. Procedures Utilized for Chronic Ligamentous Instability of the Knee, Including a Statistical Review. M.E. BLAZINA. With 4 Figures 58
    Statistical Review 58
    Description of Some Procedures 60

8. Reconstruction for Medial Instability of the Knee. Surgical Technique. D.H. O'DONOGHUE. With 8 Figures 66
    Advisability of Knee Reconstruction 66
    Surgical Technique 68
    Results 74
    Complications 74
    Conclusion 75
    References 75

9. Reconstruction of Chronic Medial Ligament Instability. S.L. JAMES. With 5 Figures 76
    Diagnosis of Instability 77
    Reconstruction Method 78
    Suggested Reading 85
    Discussion 86

10. Anterior Subluxation of the Lateral Tibial Plateau. J.C. KENNEDY 94
    Surgical Technique 95
    Common Surgical Errors 96
    Results of Surgical Treatment 97

11. Posterolateral Instability. A. TRILLAT. With 4 Figures 99
    Clinical Aspects and Examination Methods 99
    Surgical Treatment 100
    Results 103
    Discussion 103

12. Isolated Tear of the Anterior Cruciate Ligament. M.E. BLAZINA 106
    Criteria for Possible Diagnosis 106
    Possible Treatment 108

13. Prosthetic Ligaments - Indications. M.E. BLAZINA 109
    Discussion 114

Subject Index 119

List of Contributors

Dr. M.E. BLAZINA

Sherman Oaks Community Hospital
Sherman Oaks, CA 91403/USA

Dr. D.H. O'DONOGHUE

Department of Orthopaedic Surgery
The University of Oklahoma
Health Sciences Center
Oklahoma City, OK 73103/USA

Dr. S.L. JAMES

Orthopedic and Fracture
Clinic of Eugene, P.C.,
750 East 11th Ave.
Eugene, OR 97401/USA

Dr. J.C. KENNEDY

University of Western Ontario
Orthopaedic Department, Victoria Hospital
London, Ontario/Canada

Dr. A. TRILLAT

Chirurgie Orthopédique, Université de
Lyon 1, 19, Rue Montgolfier
F-69452 Lyon Cedex

Introduction

Different views about the biomechanics of the knee joint and late reconstruction of ligamentous injuries underline the obstacles impeding
the establishment of generally acceptable principles for the treatment of such lesions.

As late as June 1976, HUGHSTON emphasized in the <u>Journal of Bone and
Joint Surgery</u> that in spite of excellent anatomic studies, substantial
uncertainty still prevails in knee joint surgery. Even the significance of the anterior drawer sign for ruptures of the anterior cruciate ligament is interpreted quite diversely, as illustrated in a
comparison of HUGHSTON, GIRGIS, TORG, and SCHIECK, who give varying
opinions concerning the indication related to the age of the patient
or possible earlier joint damage as well as concerning the prognosis
for untreated knee joints. The question still remains as to how often
an intra-articular ligamentous replacement should be carried out in
addition to extra-articular techniques (O'DONOGHUE, SLOCUM, NICHOLAS,
HUGHSTON). Lastly the question of synthetic ligament replacement must
be clarified. After basic research has well advanced, clinical experience must be discussed.

Statements concerning the therapeutic value of diverse procedures
based solely on knowledge of the literature remain problematic. For
this reason a workshop was held at the University of Heidelberg in
the Orthopedic Clinic (Head: Prof. Dr. H. COTTA) in June 1977, with the
aim of bringing together representatives of the different leading
schools in a round table discussion to comment on still unsolved questions. Doctors BLAZINA, JAMES, O'DONOGHUE, and KENNEDY and Professor
TRILLAT were able to accept our invitation. The audience, composed of
delegates from western European clinics and possessing profound knowledge and experience in the field of knee joint reconstruction, was encouraged to participate in the discussions.

The main goal of the discussions was to gather detailed information
from the guest lecturers, to differentiate between their own procedures, and to carry out the different operative techniques on specimens. By the end of 1977, after the workshop was held, the American
Food and Drug Administration prohibited the use of certain synthetic
ligaments, which indicates the rapid development in this area. Some
of the contributions have therefore lost their practical, but not
their scientific, importance. Their bases are indispensable for future research.

We owe sincere gratitude to our guests, Doctor BLAZINA, Professor
O'DONOGHUE, Doctor JAMES, Professor KENNEDY, and Professor TRILLAT
for their outstanding contributions and their cooperative attitudes,
which were of great value for all participants.

We would like to express our sincere thanks to the Springer-Verlag, Heidelberg, for publishing this volume and for offering us the opportunity to pass on to others the experience of this workshop.

Heidelberg, June 1978   K.P. SCHULITZ
                                                     H. KRAHL
                                                     W.H. STEIN

1. Surgical Anatomy of the Knee

S. L. James

A discussion of knee anatomy may initially appear to be a redundant
and boring subject to the experienced orthopedic surgeon. A moment's
reflection, however, allows one to consider the importance of the
various anatomic elements particularly when approaching complicated
knee reconstructive procedures. It then becomes quite apparent that
a review of the structures which relate to the static and dynamic
stability of the knee is essential and will provide a common basis
for which to discuss complicated reconstructive ligamentous procedures.
The knee joint is the largest, most complex joint in the human body
and although its location allows easy access for examination, the diagnosis of various knee problems is often quite difficult. The proper
evaluation of knee problems is dependent upon (1) a thorough understanding of functional anatomy, (2) a systematic and orderly examination, and (3) an understanding of the various pathologic entities which
may effect the joint.

The knee is a very complicated joint allowing not only flexion and
extension but also an element of rotation and even normally some valgus
and varus motion. Knee stability is a result of both dynamic and static
elements that work as an integrated mechanism. The ligaments, capsule,
menisci, and bony contour of the joint provide static stability while
the surrounding muscles and tendons provide dynamic stability. The
static structures define the limits of motion while the musculotendinous
units control motion through voluntary and kinesthetic mechanisms. This
allows appropriate motion and simultaneously provides an energy absorbing mechanism for extrinsic and intrinsic forces which might otherwise injure the static strucutes. It is very difficult to assign a
specific function to each ligament since they work as an integrated
mechanism; attempts to do so have lead to much confusion. One must
keep in mind that rarely does an injury affect only a single element
but directly or indirectly influences one or more of the static or
dynamic structure, thus creating a complex situation for diagnosis
and treatment.

The key to evaluating ligament instability is an ability to determine
the patient's functional deficit. Two patients may have an identical
degree of ligamentous instability, but the functional deficit in each
case is not necessarily the same because of the demands which the individual may place upon the knee. One patient with a moderate amount
of instability, who desires to take part in vigorous physical activity,
may have a serious functional deficit while a more sedentary individual
may find a more severe degree of instability no serious problem what-
soever.

Medial Side of the Knee

The capsule forms somewhat of a sleeve about the knee joint, inter-
rupted anteriorly by the extensor mechanism. The medial side of the

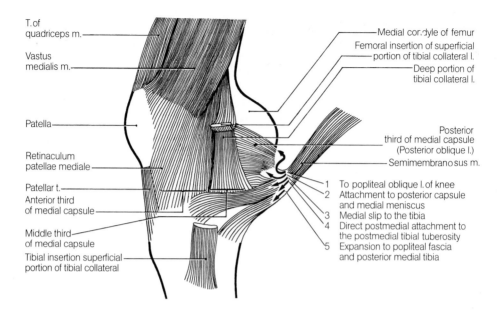

Fig. 1. Medial side of the knee. Only insertion sites of the superficial tibial collateral ligament (STCL) are shown

knee may be conveniently divided into three portions (Fig. 1). The most anterior portion consists of the anteromedial retinaculum and underlying joint capsule. It extends from the medial border of the patella and patellar tendon posteriorly to the leading edge of the superficial tibiocollateral ligament. The middle portion is referred to as the deep capsular ligament and lies deep to the superficial portion of the tibiocollateral ligament. The third or more posterior portion extends from the tibiocollateral ligament posteriorly to blend with the posterior capsule of the joint and form a sling about the medial femoral condyle. This particular portion becomes relaxed or redundant in flexion but quite tense in full extension. The posterior portion of the superficial tibiocollateral ligament (STCL) sweeps obliquely from its attachment on the femoral condyle, distally and posteriorly to attach onto the proximal portion of the tibia somewhat posteriorly and just proximal to the medial branch of the semimembranosus tendon. These fibers create a thickened portion of the medial capsule referred to as the posterior oblique ligament. This particular element is the strongest part of the medial capsule, but the STCL is the primary static stabilizing element medially and the strongest. The STCL (Fig. 2) originates from the medial aspect of the femoral condyle and sweeps distally to insert some 8-10 cm below the medial joint line on the anteromedial aspect of the proximal tibia. The anterior border consists of dense parallel collagen fibers and is quite sharply delineated. In some thin individuals this is even palpable subcutaneously. The STCL and deep capsular ligament are separated by a bursa allowing the STCL to glide back and forth with flexion and extension. Adhesions between the two structures will restrict knee motion.

The superficial and deep medial collateral ligaments stabilize the knee against excessive external rotation of the tibia as well as valgus stress. These medial structures biomechanically are in better position to resist both rotational as well as valgus forces than are the more centrally located cruciate ligaments. An acute tear of the ligamentous

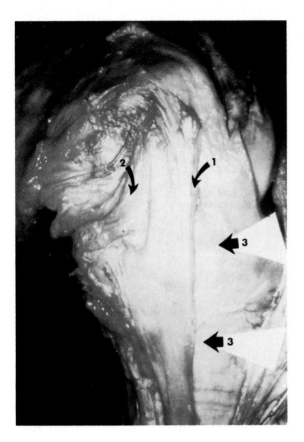

Fig. 2. The superficial tibial collateral ligament (1) dissected on a fresh specimen with the knee flexed 90°. The posterior oblique ligament (2) lies just posterior to the STCL. The larger arrows (3) indicate position of the STCL anterior margin with extension

structures medially may involve the deep capsular ligament and/or the superficial tibiocollateral ligament and in different areas from proximal to distal. Valgus and rotatory instability will occur if both the superficial and deep portions of the medial collateral ligament are torn. In this situation, however, the anterior cruciate is usually ruptured also. In some instances it is possible to have a deep capsular ligament tear, involving the midportion of the capsular ligament as well as the posterior oblique ligament, while the STCL remains intact. In this situation, the tibia will demonstrate excessive external rotation, indicative of anteromedial rotatory instability without a significant valgus component because of the intact superficial tibiocollateral ligament.

When performing reconstructive procedures medially, the surgeon should avoid attempts at repositioning the proximal insertion of the superficial tibiocollateral ligament to any significant degree. Abnormal positions of the proximal insertion may introduce large stress/strain forces on the ligaments which can subsequently create abnormal joint forces and stretch the ligamentous repair, creating additional laxity. Repositioning the distal insertion of the tibiocollateral ligament on · the other hand is less likely to create abnormal forces, and therefore it is best to reposition the ligament distally rather than proximally to avoid any significant disturbance in joint mechanics.

The semimembranosus tendon is the primary dynamic stabilizing element on the posteromedial aspect of the knee. Most textbooks of anatomy fail

to mention the several branches of this tendon and don't emphasize its
dynamic stabilizing function. One branch of the semimembranosus tendon
passes lateral, blending into the posterior capsule to form the oblique
popliteal ligament, which is a heavy ligamentous structure crossing the
posterior capsule obliquely to insert above the lateral femoral condyle
in the area of the lateral head of the gastrocnemius insertion. Another branch attaches directly to the posterior capsule and the posterior rim of the medial meniscus, allowing some dynamic control of
the medial meniscus by retracting it somewhat posteriorly. A third
portion is a tendinous-like structure which passes medially along the
proximal tibia to attach deep to the STCL. This is the portion which
is classically shown in anatomy textbooks, and one often has the impression that this is the only insertion of the semimembranosus tendon.
Another part inserts directly into the posterior medial tibial tuberosity and a fifth expansion passes distally, blending into the popliteal fascia. The semimembranosus tendon can be utilized to reinforce
the posterior medial aspect of the knee by reefing it into the repair
site in acute or reconstructive procedures.

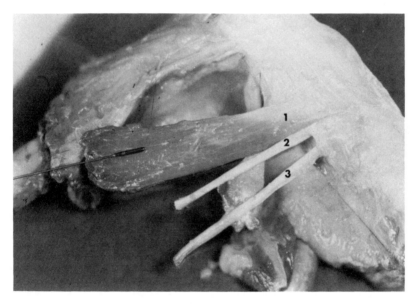

Fig. 3. The pes anserinus with the sartorius (1), the gracilis (2), and semitendinosus
tendons (3)

Medially, the sartorius, gracilis and semitendinosus muscles form a
structure called the pes anserinus (Fig. 3). The sartorius lies most
proximal and the semitendinosus most distal with the gracilis located
between them. The insertion of these three tendons forms a web-like
structure referred to as the pes anserinus or "goose-foot." It is this
structure which Dr. DONALD SLOCUM has utilized in the pes anserinus
transplant. The most important element is the semitendinosus or distal
most portion of the pes anserinus. The effectiveness of the pes anserinus transplant is dependent upon a more proximal and anterior repositioning of the semitendinosus under the medial flare of the tibia.
The most common mistake made in performing a pes anserinus transplant
is failure to include the semitendinosus tendon.

A structure related to the pes anserinus which must be considered in doing the pes anserinus transplant, is the sartorial branch of the saphenous nerve. This small nerve exists distally between the sartorius and gracilis muscles and supplies sensation to the anteromedial aspect of the leg. It has no motor function, but damaging this structure during the course of a pes anserinus transplant can create a disturbing area of hypesthesia for the patient.

In instances where the medial capsular and ligamentous structures have been severely attenuated, the sartorius may be transferred obliquely across the medial aspect of the joint; it should be left attached distally and secured more proximally along the posterior margin of the vastus medialis oblique muscle which dynamically reinforces the deficient medial ligaments. In addition to this, the vastus medialis obliquus may be advanced distally and posteriorly to further reinforce the deficient medial structures.

In summary, we find that the medial side of the knee joint is stabilized by both static and dynamic structures. The static stabilizing structures are (1) the medial capsule, (2) the deep and superficial tibiocollateral ligaments, (3) the cruciate ligaments, (4) the medial portion of the posterior capsule, (5) the medial meniscus, and (6) the bony contour of the femoral condyle and the tibial plateau.

The dynamic medial stabilizing structures are (1) the vastus medialis obliquus muscle, (2) the pes anserinus muscles (sartorius, gracilis and semitendinosus), (3) the semimembranosus muscle with its many ramifications, and (4) the medial head of the gastrocnemius. All of these structures are not truly located on the medial side of the knee, but they do contribute to medial joint stability.

Posterior Structures of the Knee

The most significant structures posteriorly are (1) the posterior capsule, (2) the oblique popliteal ligament, (3) arcuate ligament, (4) the popliteus muscle, and (5) the medial and lateral gastrocnemius tendons (Fig. 4).

The oblique popliteal ligament was mentioned previously and was found to be formed by one branch of the semimembranosus tendon. It is a heavy ligamentous thickening of the posterior capsule passing obliquely from medial to lateral across the posterior aspect of the joint. It becomes tense when the semimembranosus contracts and quite likely serves a significant stabilizing effect on the knee via the semimembranosus muscle. The exact role and function of the posterior oblique ligament is at this time still not fully understood. Posteriorly and laterally, the capsule arches over the popliteus muscle, forming the arcuate ligament which continues laterally to insert on to the fibular styloid. The arcuate ligament is one part of the arcuate complex referred to in reconstructive surgery consisting of the arcuate ligament, the popliteus tendon, and the lateral collateral ligament. These elements form an essential entity in reconstructive procedures for posterolateral and anterolateral instability of the knee.

The popliteus muscle takes origin from the posterior, proximal aspect of the tibia and is oriented somewhat obliquely, running proximally and laterally. The medial two-thirds of the popliteus insert into the arcuate ligament or posterior capsule as well as the posterior horn of the lateral meniscus. The lateral one-third of the popliteus muscle

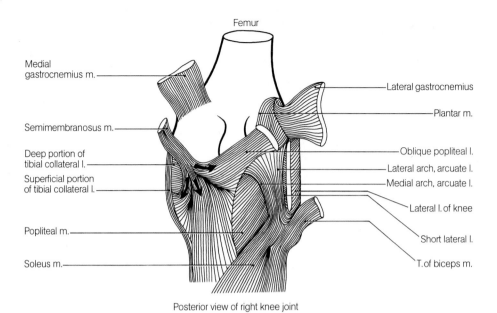

Medial gastrocnemius m.

Lateral gastrocnemius

Plantar m.

Semimembranosus m.

Deep portion of tibial collateral l.

Superficial portion of tibial collateral l.

Oblique popliteal l.

Lateral arch, arcuate l.

Medial arch, arcuate l.

Lateral l. of knee

Popliteal m.

Short lateral l.

Soleus m.

T. of biceps m.

Posterior view of right knee joint

Fig. 4. Posterior view of right knee joint

becomes a definite tendinous structure, passing along the lateral femoral condyle under the fibular collateral ligament to insert on to the lateral femoral condyle. The popliteus muscle is primarily an internal rotator of the tibia in relation to the femur, but it also prevents forward displacement of the femur on the tibia during flexion of the knee. Electromyographically, the popliteus becomes very active during normal walking from about the midportion of the swing phase, at which time the tibia is internally rotating on the femur through most of the stance phase. The tibia internally rotates in the early stance phase in relation to the femur as a result of foot pronation in the subtalar joint which creates an obligatory internal tibial rotation. This position of the tibia is maintained in relation to the femur by activity of the popliteus muscle. Repositioning the insertion of the popliteus tendon on the lateral femoral condyle more proximally and anteriorly is one of the steps in reconstructive surgery for posterior lateral rotatory instability.

The posterior capsule provides a significant degree of knee stability with the knee in full extension. In this position, all the remaining ligamentous structures can be disrupted, but with the knee forced into full extension, no medial or lateral instability will be apparent. This is important clinically in assessing collateral ligamentous laxity. The knee must be flexed slightly in order to relax the posterior capsule to determine accurately the integrity of the collateral ligaments. If the posterior capsule has been ruptured, it is also quite likely that the posterior cruciate ligament has been involved to some extent. Likewise, it is unlikely that an injury is confined to the posterior structures without involving either the posterior medial or posterior lateral structures as well.

The medial and lateral heads of the gastrocnemius insert above their respective femoral condyles. The medial gastrocnemius has a longer, more definite tendinous configuration and can be used as a substitute in reconstructive procedures for the posterior cruciate ligament. The medial head can be released and passed through the posterior capsule into the notch of the femur to be attached at the original insertion of the posterior cruciate ligament. The lateral tendon of the gastrocnemius is frequently transferred anteriorly to help tighten the posterior capsule with posterolateral instabilities. The tendon of the lateral gastrocnemius blends with the posterior capsule at the insertion above the lateral femoral condyle, and consequently migrating the tendon of the gastrocnemius anteriorly along the lateral femoral condyle will tighten the posterior capsule as well. This procedure is frequently combined with an anterior advancement of the proximal insertion of fibular collateral ligament and the popliteus tendon.

Lateral Structures

The lateral side of the knee is also stabilized by dynamic and static elements. The static stabilizers laterally are (1) the iliotibial tract, (2) the fibular collateral ligament, (3) the lateral one-half of the posterior capsule, (4) the arcuate ligament, (5) the cruciate ligaments, and (6) the lateral meniscus. Dynamic stabilizing structures laterally are (1) the biceps muscle, (2) the popliteus muscle, (3) the lateral head of the gastrocnemius, and (4) the vastus lateralis. By this time it should be apparent to the reader that there is considerable overlap in the function of the various structures and that arbitrarily assigning them to the medial, posterior, or lateral side of the knee is purely a matter of convenience for discussion.

Static stress testing on postmortum specimens suggests that the fibular collateral ligament provides the primary resistance against varus stress, but the iliotibial tract, the popliteus muscle, and ramifications of the biceps tendon also play a very significant role in lateral stability. The fibular collateral ligament is a rather small, tendon-like structure, extending from the lateral femoral condyle distally to insert on to the head of the fibula, and it seems quite unlikely that this small, rather tenuous structure alone is the primary static stabilizer against varus instability. The clinical significance of the fibular collateral ligament is that when it is ruptured, it signifies that there has been a significant injury to the other lateral stabilizing structures as well.

The iliotibial tract is an important static stabilizing element and perhaps also has some dynamic function via the tensor fascia lata. Proximally it has some attachment to the intermuscular septum at the level of the lateral femoral epicondyle. It passes across the lateral aspect of the joint to insert distally onto the anterolateral aspect of the proximal tibia to an area referred to as Gerdy's tubercle. The iliotibial tract glides back and forth with flexion and extension of the knee.

The midlateral capsule is easily palpable between the posterior edge of the iliotibial tract and the fibular collateral ligament. This structure is a rather thin, filmy element which quite likely does have some lateral stabilizing effect but does not appear to be a major stabilizing element. HUGHSTON has emphasized the role of the midlateral capsule in stabilizing the knee and suggests that injury to this structure plays a significant role in developing anterolateral rotatory instability. I personally have seen this structure torn in acute ligament injuries in which there was a positive McIntosh sign indicative of anterolateral rotatory instability of the "pivot-shift" type. The midlateral capsule probably does play a role in anterolateral rotatory instability, but the primary lesion in this entity seems to be incompetency of the anterior cruciate ligament with a more secondary involvement of the midlateral capsule.

The vastus lateralis muscle is somewhat analogous to the vastus medialis obliquus medially, but it does not influence patellar function as significantly. Its fibers terminate more proximal than do the vastus medialis obliquus fibers and are more longitudinally oriented as opposed to the more oblique fibers of the vastus medialis which very directly control the patella and stabilize it against lateral displacement.

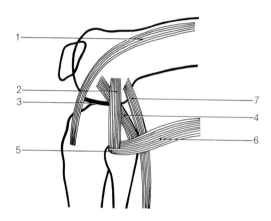

Fig. 5. Lateral side of the knee. The iliotibial tract (1) crosses the joint anteriorly to insert on Gerdy's tubercle. The midlateral capsule between the iliotibial tract and fibular collateral ligament (2) has been excised, exposing the lateral meniscus (3). The popliteus tendon (4) lies immediately behind the fibular collateral ligament. The superficial portion of the biceps tendon insertion (5) attaches to the tibia anterior to the fibular head while the middle layer (6) encompasses the distal insertion of the fibular collateral ligament. The lateral head of the gastrocnemius (7) passes proximally to its insertion above the lateral femoral condyle

The most important lateral stabilizing structure dynamically is the biceps muscle (Fig. 5), which is somewhat analogous to the semimembranosus muscle, medially. Functionally the biceps is a flexor of the knee and external rotator of the tibia on the femur. The biceps insertion has three layers with the superficial layer extending somewhat anteriorly to attach onto the lateral aspect of the proximal tibia anterior to the fibula. The midportion of the tendon envelopes the distal insertion of the fibular collateral ligament and attaches to the posterior aspect of the fibular collateral ligament. A deeper element spans the space between the fibula to the posterolateral aspect of the tibia and capsule.

It has an expansion to the iliotibial tract which tightens the iliotibial tract upon contraction, and its expansion to the posterior capsule helps tense the posterior capsule. This structure dynamically has a considerable amount of control posteriorly and laterally. The tendon of the biceps may be utilized as a dynamic reinforcement for lateral instabilities, but one should not dissect out the deep expansion between the tibia and fibula because of its important dynamic and static stabilization effect on the lateral side of the knee.

Unfortunately there is no single well-defined structure laterally that can be indicated as a primary static stabilizing element as there is medially. Reconstructive procedures on the lateral side of the knee are subsequently somewhat ambiguous and perhaps not as clearly delineated as on the medial side.

It has been mentioned earlier in this paper that the bony contour of the knee joint plays a role in stability. The medial tibial plateau is somewhat dish-shaped or slightly concave, while the lateral plateau of the tibia is more convex and does not present a flat surface to the femoral condyle. Posteriorly, the lateral tibial plateau drops off rather acutely, and the articular cartilage continues down over the posterior lip of the plateau. The lateral meniscus is retracted posteriorly by the popliteus and slides onto this particular area of the plateau with knee flexion. The topography and contour of the lateral plateau most likely plays a role in the mechanics of anterolateral rotatory instability referred to as the "pivot-shift" by MACINTOSH. With incompetency of the anterior cruciate ligament, the lateral femoral condyle is allowed to glide more posteriorly on the convex surface of the lateral plateau, allowing it to become momentarily impinged in this position until reduced by tightening of the iliotibial tract with knee flexion.

Cruciate Ligaments

The cruciate ligaments are incredibly complex structures both architecturally and functionally. They are intra-articular but extrasynovial (Fig. 6). The anterior cruciate ligament arises from the tibia, courses posteriorly, superiorly, and laterally to insert on to the lateral femoral condyle in a crescentric fashion oriented somewhat obliquely

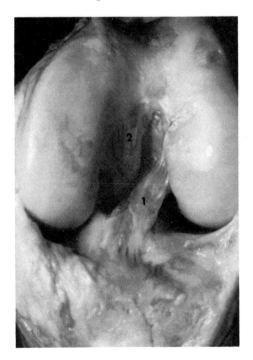

Fig. 6. Cruciate ligaments. The anterior cruciate ligament (1) passes from anterior on the tibia proximally and posteriorly to insert on the medial aspect of the lateral femoral condyle. Femoral insertion of the posterior cruciate ligament (2) attaches well anterior and superior in the notch. The knee is flexed 90°, with the anterior cruciate oriented more horizontally and the posterior cruciate more vertically

but for the most part vertically with the knee in extension. The insertion is far posterior and high in the notch near the articular margin of the lateral femoral condyle. Lying behind the anterior cruciate ligament is the larger and bulkier posterior cruciate ligament which passes anteriorly and obliquely from its origin on the tibia posteriorly to insert onto the lateral aspect of the medial femoral condyle anteriorly and high in the notch area, again close to the articular margin of the medial femoral condyle. Its femoral attachment is also crescentric in shape but oriented more horizontally with the knee in extension. The orientation of the insertion on the femoral condyles of both cruciate ligaments changes dramatically as the knee passes from extension to flexion. This creates a reciprocal tightness or tenseness within various portions of each ligament at all degrees of flexion.

It is important to remember that the anterior cruciate ligament is covered with a layer of synovium. If the synovium remains intact following acute injury, the anterior cruciate ligament may appear to be grossly intact. Incising the synovium to further inspect the cruciate ligament may reveal the extent of the injury, however; a normal appearing cruciate ligament can be totally incompetent due to interstitial tearing of the ligament which is not apparent grossly.

The complex architecture of the cruciate ligaments has made replacement of these structures by a prosthetic ligament extremely difficult. The fibers of the anterior cruciate, for instance, are largely oriented longitudinally, but they also spiral from one insertion site to the other so that the geometry of the ligament is difficult to duplicate by artificial means.

The function of the cruciate ligaments is quite complex and has been very confusing, with numerous reports from various investigators. There definitely appears to be some reciprocity between the anterior and posterior cruciate ligaments in flexion and extension so that some elements do remain tight or tense in all positions and thus provide some stability regardless of knee position. This factor again makes artificial substitution a most difficult task.

Although the cruciate ligaments do play a significant role in stabilizing the medial and lateral side of the knee, biomechanically they are not positioned as effectively as are the collateral ligaments in resisting rotatory or varus/valgus forces. They are better positioned to resist forces in the sagittal plane. Their specific function is difficult to describe thoroughly because it cannot be isolated from the other ligamentous structures about the knee. The anterior cruciate ligament certainly stabilizes the tibia from anterior displacement in relation to the femoral condyles and also stabilizes the knee against hyperextension. There are, however, instances noted at surgery in which the anterior cruciate ligament has been totally ruptured without a significant anterior drawer sign being evident clinically. In this instance the collateral structures provide sufficient stability to prevent anterior displacement of the tibia. The posterior cruciate ligament prevents posterior displacement or subluxation of the tibial plateaus in relation to the femoral condyles. The posterior drawer sign may not be present with acute posterior cruciate rupture if the posterior medial and lateral structures have remained intact. In chronic situations, however, a positive posterior drawer sign not only indicates incompetency or absence of the posterior cruciate ligament but also attenuation of the posterior lateral and posterior medial structures as well. HUGHSTON has indicated that the posterior cruciate ligament will also allow anterior shift of the tibia or, in other words, an anterior drawer sign. This has also been verified in the laboratory by MAINS et al.

Statically, the cruciate ligaments have a tendency to relax with external tibial rotation and tighten with internal tibial rotation. Even without an anterior cruciate ligament the posterior cruciate ligament becomes quite tight with internal tibial rotation and stabilizes the knee by pulling the joint surfaces together. Thus, with an intact posterior cruciate ligament there is no abnormal motion of the tibia with drawer test when the tibia is internally rotated when doing the Slocum test. However, when the tibia is placed into external rotation and the anterior cruciate ligament is incompetent, the posterior cruciate ligament does not stabilize the knee, and a positive sign for anteromedial rotatory instability with a positive drawer sign is present with the Slocum test.

Menisci

The menisci are two semilunar shaped pieces of fibrocartilage which have a peripheral attachment to the adjacent tissues by coronary ligaments. The medial meniscus is larger and C-shaped while the lateral meniscus is smaller and more oval in configuration. Laterally the inferior geniculate artery runs within the substance of the coronary ligament and is easily cut during the course of lateral meniscectomy. The medial meniscus is firmly attached about the periphery and is closely adherent to the deep capsular ligament but is not directly attached to the superficial tibiocollateral ligament. The medial meniscus is less mobile than the lateral meniscus and more subject to injury, particularly posterior-medially where it is thickest and widest. The lateral meniscus on the other hand is not as firmly attached about its periphery and is more mobile, which probably accounts for the fact that it is less frequently injured. Both menisci slide posteriorly with flexion and are thrust forward by the femoral condyles as the knee extends. The lateral meniscus is under dynamic control of the popliteus muscle which retracts it posteriorly with knee flexion. The semimembranosus retracts the medial meniscus posteriorly with flexion but to a much lesser extent due to its more secure fixation to the surrounding soft tissues. Both menisci have tibial attachments at their anterior and posterior horns in the intercondylar area of the tibial plateaus. The posterior horn of the lateral meniscus sometimes has two additional attachments to the lateral aspect of the medial femoral condyle. One is the ligament of WRISBERG which lies on the posterior aspect of the posterior cruciate ligament somewhat paralleling the posterior cruciate ligament and is present in about 60%-70% of knees. Another small ligament, called the ligament of HUMPHREY, occasionally lies anterior to the posterior cruciate ligament, again taking origin from the posterior horn of the lateral meniscus and attaching to the medial femoral condyle anterior to the posterior cruciate ligament. It is unusual to find both ligaments present in the same knee. Perhaps these small ligaments act as restraints while guiding motion of the posterior horn of the lateral meniscus.

For quite some time it was felt that the menisci served no significant function and were expendable. More recent studies, however, have indicated that this is not true. The menisci increase the joint contact area between the femur and tibia and also have a significant weight-bearing role. Without a meniscus, weight-bearing forces are concentrated over a smaller area, encouraging degenerative changes. In addition to their weight-bearing role, the menisci also enhance knee stability. It is not unusual to find increased anteromedial rotatory instability of the knee following removal of the medial meniscus which eliminates the stabilizing effect of the posterior horn. The menisci are not to

be thought of as ancillary elements in the knee which can be discarded
with little regard.

This has been a rather brief, superficial summary of knee anatomy. Its
importance cannot be overemphasized in regard to knee ligament surgery.
The reader is strongly encouraged to refer to the list of suggested
reading for more details.

Suggested Reading

1. SARTELL, D.L. et al.: Surgical repositioning of the medial collateral ligament.
   J. Bone Joint Surg. 59A, 107 (Jan 1977)
2. BASMAJIAN, J.V. et al.: Functions of the popliteus muscle in Man. J. Bone Joint
   Surg. 53A, 557 (April 1971)
3. ENGIN, A.E., KORDE, M.S.: Biomechanics of normal and abnormal knee joint. J.
   Biomech. 7, 325-335 (1977)
4. FEAGIN, J.L. et al.: Isolated tear of the anterior cruciate ligament: 5-Year
   follow up study. Am. J. Sports Med. 4, 95-100 (May/Jun 1976)
5. GIRGIS, F.G. et al.: The cruciate ligaments of the knee joint. Anatomical,
   functional and experimental analysis. Clin. Orthop. 106, 216-231 (1975)
6. HARTY, M.: Anatomic features of the lateral aspect of the knee. SGO 130, 11
   (Jan 1970)
7. HUGHSTON, J.C. et al.: The role of the posterior oblique ligament in repairs of
   acute medial (collateral) ligament tears of the knee. J. Bone Joint Surg. 55A,
   923 (July 1973)
8. KAPLAN, E.B.: Iliotibial Tract. J. Bone Joint Surg. 40A, 817 (1958)
9. KARPF, P.M.: Anatomic principals as a prerequisite for the diagnosis of knee
   ligament injuries in skiing. Fortschr. Med. 95, 191 (Jan 1977)
10. KENNEDY, J.C. et al.: The anatomy and function of the anterior cruciate ligament.
    J. Bone Joint Surg. 56A, 223 (March 1974)
11. KENNEDY, J.C., FOWLER, P.J.: Medial and anterior instability of the knee. J.
    Bone Joint Surg. 53A, 1257 (1971)
12. KETTLEKAMP, D.: An electrogoniometric study of knee joint motion in normal gait.
    J. Bone Joint Surg. 52A, 775 (1970)
13. LANGA, G.S.: Experimental observations and interpretations on the relationship
    between the morphology and function of the human knee joint. Acta Anat. 55,
    16-38 (1963)
14. MCLOED, W.D. et al.: Tibial plateau topography. Am. J. Sports Med. 5, 13 (1977)
15. MAINS, D.B., ANDREWS, J.G., STONCIPHER, T.: Medial and anterior-posterior liga-
    ment stability of the human knee, measured with a stress apparatus. Am. J. Sports
    Med. 5, 144-153 (1977)
16. MANN, R.A. et al.: The popliteus muscle. J. Bone Joint Surg. 59A, 924 (Oct 1977)
17. MARSHALL, J.L. et al.: The biceps femoris tendon and its functional significance.
    J. Bone Joint Surg. 54A, 1440 (Oct 1972)
18. MORRISON, J.B.: The mechanics of the knee joint in relation to normal walking.
    J. Biomech. 3, 51 (1970)
19. NOYES, F.R. et al.: Biomechanical function of the pes anserinus at the knee and
    the effect of its transplantation. J. Bone Joint Surg. 55A, 1225 (Sep 1973)
20. NOYES, F.R. et al.: The strength of the anterior cruciate ligament in human and
    rhesus monkeys. J. Bone Joint Surg. 58A, 1074-1082 (Dec. 1976)
21. O'DONOGHUE, D.H.: Reconstruction for medical instability of the knee. J. Bone
    Joint Surg. 55A, 941 (1973)
22. PALMER, I.: On injuries to the ligaments of the knee joint. Acta Chir. Scandinav.
    (Suppl. 53) 81, 3-282 (1938)
23. SLOCUM, D.B. et al.: Pes anserinus transplantation. J. Bone Joint Surg. 50A,
    226 (March 1968)
24. SLOCUM, D.B. et al.: Rotary instability of the knee. J. Bone Joint Surg. 50A,
    211 (March 1968)
25. SLOCUM, D.B., JAMES, S.L.: Athletic injuries of the lower extremity. Orthopedic
    Digest, p. 15-31 (Jun 1977)

26. SLOCUM, D.B., LARSON, R.L., JAMES, S.L.: Late reconstruction of ligamentous in-
    juries of the medial compartment of the knee. Clin. Orthop. No. 100, pp. 23-55
    (May 1974)
27. SLOCUM, D.B., LARSON, R.L., JAMES, S.L.: Pes anserinus transplant: impressions
    after a decade of experience. J. Sports Med. 2, 123-136 (May/Jun 1974)
28. WARREN, L.F. et al.: The prime static stabilizer of the medial side of the knee.
    J. Bone Joint Surg. 56A, 665 (Jun 1974)

Discussion

TRILLAT: The movements of the two menisci have been studied. The internal meniscus is only slightly displaced in flexion. This backward
displacement does not exceed 1.5 cm.

As soon as there is a movement of the tibia in an external abduction
rotation, the internal meniscus is pulled towards the interior of the
joint and can completely luxate when the peripheral capsular structures have been suppressed. This is the same displacement which occurs
when there is a lesion of the internal meniscus in a bucket-handle
lesion.

In an inversed maneuver on the tibia, one can achieve replacement of
the luxated bucket-handle in the intercondylar fossa.

As far as the lateral meniscus is concerned, everything is more complex
because of the large, almost circular development of this cartilage.
It seems to be the center of the rotational movements of the tibia on
the femur. Its backward displacement in the movement from complete
extension to flexion is much more important than that of the internal
meniscus - practically twice as important. This explains first of all
that there is frequently a lesion in the movement from flexion to
extension. This also explains that in extension, its anterior horn,
often very large, will be laminated and has therefore undergone a
trauma. This is not the case with the anterior horn of the internal
meniscus which is only torn if there is a posterior gap as well.

SCHULITZ: Dr. JAMES, what is the importance of the Humphrey and the
Wrisberg ligaments?

JAMES: The ligament of Wrisberg lies behind the posterior cruciate
ligament, is attached to the posterior horn of the lateral meniscus,
runs parallel to the course of the posterior cruciate ligament, and
is attched to the medial femoral condyle. The ligament of Humphrey
follows it in a somewhat similar course but lies in front of the
posterior cruciate ligament. The exact function of these ligaments
is not quite clear, but they probably act as a control device for
motion of the lateral meniscus.

THIEL: You said something about the important role of the meniscus
for the nutrition of the knee.

JAMES: The nutrition of the articular cartilage of the knee depends
primarily upon the synovial fluid. The role of the meniscus is not
primarily that of nutrition, the nutrition probably being due to
compression and relaxation of the articular cartilage. But the menisci do help spread the synovial fluid throughout the knee joint and
in that way do help protect the supply of nutrition to the articular

cartilage by coating them constantly with synovial fluid. Since they are of some importance for the weight-bearing function, they help in nutrition of articular cartilage.

STEIN: I would like to point out one thing which has been emphasized by the group of WARREN/GIRGIS/MARSHALL, and that is the differentiation of the anterior cruciate into two subportions: the so-called anteromedial band and the posterior portion. These have a different significance for the internal and external rotatory stability of the knee joint.

JAMES: In a recent work WARREN, GIRGIS, and MARSHALL indicated that the anterior cruciate ligament does have two portions, as well as the posterior cruciate ligament. I think that needs more clarification. I personally do not feel that this small portion, the anteromedial portion of the anterior cruciate ligament, can be disrupted without some damage to the rest of the ligament also. And I also think that it relates to the fact that what we grossly see in the knee joint at the time of an acute knee injury does not always reflect what is actually going to occur from a functional standpoint. Granted, we may see that the anterior medial portion as they described has been ruptured, but in fact there is probably likewise some damage to the core of the anterior cruciate ligament that can only be seen microscopically get will prohibit normal functioning.

SCHULITZ: Is there a difference between the lateral head of the semimembranosus and the posterior oblique ligament?

JAMES: The branch or portion of the semimembranosus which passes posteriorly into the posterior capsule is called the oblique popliteal ligament. This is not to be confused with the posterior oblique ligament which HUGHSTON has described. The posterior oblique ligament in the old literature was referred to as the superior oblique fibers of the tibicollateral ligament. So the posterior oblique ligament is a portion of the tibiocollateral ligament, while the oblique popliteal ligament is a portion of the posterior capsule. I know that these terms are rather confusing, but they are different anatomic structures.

BRUSSATIS: There are different opinions about what the tibia does when the knee joint is extended. Some say there is an external rotation. What is correct?

JAMES: The question is what type of tibial rotation occurs passively with flexion and extension of the knee. With passive or active extension of the knee the tibia externally rotates in relation to the femoral condyles, and with flexion it internally rotates. The confusion arises because of the reference point of rotation. In some references the rotation is described with the tibia stationary and the femoral condyles rotating in relation to the tibia. In others the rotation is described with the femoral condyles remaining stationary and the tibia rotating. I think that is where the confusion arises. The actual fact is that in relation to the femoral condyles the tibia externally rotates normally with extension and internally rotates with flexion.

MÜLLER: Already in the last century a medial collateral ligament and a posterior medial collateral ligament were described. I found an ancient preparation of a so-called medial collateral ligament in our institute and determined that it was that very portion of the medial collateral ligament now known as the Hughston posterior oblique ligament. I think the meniscus is maximally fixed by the ligament structures in just this area of the posterior oblique ligament because chronic disruptions of the meniscus begin in this area. I personally do not agree with Dr. JAMES in that this ligament slacks in flexion. This part still functions very well on the medial side in extension and also in flexion. I first tried to restore these structures in fresh lesions in all my knee ligament reconstructions. Then, however, I found that if there are quite well sutured, there is practically no more medial instability.

JAMES: This is the same part of the tibiocollateral ligament which BRANTIGAN and VOSHELL described way back in the forties as the superior oblique fibers of the tibiocollateral ligament. Consequently, it is not a new structure anatomically. It has been described. HUGHSTON broke it down into three elements. I feel this element is somewhat relaxed with knee flexion although it is a heavier, denser portion of the capsule which you can feel. To get into the posterior compartment of the knee joint, you must have the incision just along the trailing edge of the structure to allow adequate retraction. This is the area where the repairs must be undertaken.

SCHULITZ: Is the anterior cruciate ligament at 90° flexion tight or slack?

As you know, HUGHSTON has a different interpretation. Could you please clarify this?

KENNEDY: Our studies have shown that the anterior cruciate ligament is reasonably slack at 90°. It is starting to approach tightness, but from about 45°-70° of flexion it is lax. As it approaches full flexion at 90°, 100°, and 120° it starts to get tight. If at 90 you internally rotate the tibia on the femur it will then become tight.

SCHULITZ: Do you not agree with HUGHSTON?

KENNEDY: Not in that, nor in many other things.

MOSCHI: Do you have any information in vivo, not in vitro, that the menisci do bear weight, because if they do, then the point that Dr. TRILLAT made that the posterior horn of the medial meniscus is the one most often damaged could not be maintained. However, I really believe what Dr. TRILLAT says about the posterior horn being the part most often damaged in the medial meniscus; this would conform with actual information from electrokinesiology. The periphery of the meniscus gives information on the status in the space of the medial condyle during flexion. If a part of the posterior horn is apart from the insertion of the semimembranosous, this would give less stimulus to the semimembranosus to pull the meniscus backwards during flexion.

KENNEDY: That is a very interesting concept. I don't have any facts to back up this theory, but I think that the kinesthetic feedback to the knee joint is a very important element, particularly when we consider rehabilitation and restoration of function. Perhaps many of the failures that we have in reconstructive surgery are actually failures of restoration of the kinesthetic system of the knee joint. We have done some studies on nerve supply to the menisci and cruciate ligaments, and they both seem to have a nerve supply. The nerve cell looks as if it may conduct proprioceptive sensations from that area and has a sense of positive in humans.

KRAHL: If there are different opinions as to the state of tension of the anterior cruciate ligament in flexion, I wonder if there is a certain anterior drawer sign in an isolated tear of the anterior cruciate ligament?

JAMES: In North America it is becoming more and more decided that there is really no such thing as an isolated tear of the anterior cruciate ligament. Dr. BLAZINA may differ slightly with this though I doubt it. We feel that in most tears of the anterior cruciate ligament there will be at least some microscopic damage to the lateral and medial corners of the knee joint and that subsequently they will begin to function in deficit: as a result, we think that you can go in and see a torn anterior cruciate ligament where the anterior drawer sign is for quite some time not positive. If, however, you follow any of these cases as we have for 7-10 years, we feel you will concur with our opinion that a slow progression of difficulties follows which eventually leads to trouble.

SCHULITZ: What do think about the Lachmann sign?

KENNEDY: This sign is done with the knee almost in extension when testing the anterior drawer sign. I think it can be helpful. The determination of an anterior drawer sign should be done in neutral position, in external and internal rotation, and then in varying degrees of flexion to extension. Every position gives a little more information. Perhaps this may be the sign that eventually determines whether the posterior lateral or anterior medial fibers of the cruciate ligament are involved.

STEIN: I would like to mention again the very essential work of MARSHALL and GIRGIS, pointing out that in 90° flexion of the knee joint the anteromedial band of the anterior cruciate is tight. This probably will be the determining factor of the anterior drawer sign, whereas the bulk of the anterior cruciate in 90° flexion is relaxed. Furthermore, as Dr. KENNEDY already said, in 1941 BRANTIGAN and VOSHELL (and in 1911 the German anatomist FICK) showed that during nearly all degrees of flexion of the knee joint some portion of either the anterior cruciate or the posterior cruciate is tense. This might explain to a certain degree the difficulties in defining the anterior and posterior drawer sign in knee joint injuries. I would like to cite MARSHALL, who stated that in nearly 90% of the isolated anterior cruciate ruptures which he operated, he found a positive anterior drawer sign.

2. Biomechanics of the Ligaments of the Knee

J.C. Kennedy

Our studies on tension in ligaments above the knee joint are actually
microscopic determinations; we elected to evaluate by laboratory studies the failing strength of ligaments, as well as the relative strains,
and the position of the knee joint in which the ligament is most taut.
We felt the need to delineate the properties of ligaments, which we
did by first comparing the ultimate failing strength when the ligament totally failed. We then compared it to the structure under microscope of these ligaments just before they failed and after they failed.

Method of Measurement

We used what we call an instron tension analyser and adapted it to
study the tensile properties of the three ligaments in the knee joint.
Often you get slippage of the clamps, so we modified the tension analyser to have rather coarse clamp serrations to prevent slippage of
the ligament.

We initially tested ten anterior cruciates, ten posterior cruciates,
and ten tibiocollateral ligaments. The entire ligament was excised
from each joint less than 12 hours after death, and all were tested on
an instron analyser within 4 hours from time of removal. These ligaments were fixed only in saline and were suspended from the upper portion of the clamp and hung freely in order to accept their own orientation. Then each ligament was subjected to an increasing load, gradually
building up to several hundred kg. Initially we tested at a rate of
12.5 cm/min and then repeated the same tests at what we now consider
possible physiological loading at 50 cm/min. We repeated these tests
on ten more ligaments of each type until a total number of 60 ligaments
had been tested. A scanning electron microscope was then utilized to
study the internal fibrillar collagen arrangement of such ligaments
before and after the extension tests. Specimens that we took from the
midportion of each ligament were 1 cm long, about 3 mm wide, and 3 mm
deep. The first group of ligaments was taken from the exact midportion
of five anterior, five posterior, and five tibiocollateral ligaments
that had not been stressed. These were just normal sections. Then we
obtained similar tests and similar specimens from 15 more ligaments
which had been stressed just to the joint of failure but had not visibly
ruptured; finally, a third group with actual visible disruption was
removed and tested.

In these ligaments we were chiefly interested in two determinations:
the ultimate failure point, the point beyond which the ligament can
support no or only a negligible load, and the physiological loading
rate by which a ligament fails. Here is a descriptive example; a ligament loaded at a slow rate (0.5 cm/min) grossly looks intact at the
point at which the instron measures failure. From this point until
visible destruction becomes evident, the ligament is not producing
any resistance to stress (i.e., it fails), yet only upon microscopic
examination can one see evidence of failure. Then, at the point of

final rupture, there is gross visible destruction of fibers within the ligament.

Laboratory Testing and Results

In studying these ligaments, we found that 20 anterior cruciates and 20 tibiocollateral ligaments had almost equal failing strengths, whereas the posterior cruciate ligaments failed at almost twice the value of the other ligaments. I think this is important to remember because it emphasizes the importance of the posterior cruciate ligament, of which the resistance in the knee joint is twice that of the anterior cruciate or the tibiocollateral ligament.

We feel that most knee ligaments failed clinically under rather fast loading rates. However, since in our country and in our continent the exact physiological loading rate by which a ligament fails has never been accurately determined, we were interested in attempting this. We felt that 12.5 was really too slow a loading rate, and yet interestingly enough at 12.5 cm/min and at 50 cm/min, the posterior cruciate ligament still maintains about the same ratio of being twice as strong as the other two ligaments. As you may know, what we describe as viscoelastic properties have been shown in animal; our experiments show that human ligaments behave similarly, absorbing more energy and requiring more force to rupture as the loading rate is increased. The final rupture of the tibiocollateral ligament in this study occurred at 46.3 kg at a loading rate of only 12.5 cm/min, and yet it was raised to 67.8 kg when the loading rate was increased to 50 cm/min. In other words, the faster the loading rate, the more force is required to rupture the ligament.

In the past the bone-ligament preparation has been described as the best method of studying tensile properties in ligaments. However, we concur more with the recent publications which indicate that the failure is usually not at the bone-ligament interface and that the faster the loading rate, the more likely the failure is to be in the intraligamentous portion. The weakest link in the chain is the intraligamentous portion of this complex, particularly when the loading rate is rapid. Our clinical observations in a small series of what Dr. BLAZINA would call isolated tears showed that some 72% of our anterior cruciate tears were in the midsubstance of the ligament, whereby we described the midportion as the middle half of an overall 4 cm long ligament, i.e., the middle 2 cm.

Moving on to our studies using the scanning electron microscope, we observed both the cruciate and the tibiocollateral ligament. A normal dog's cruciate ligament tested at 50 cm/min could illustrate Dr. JAMES' statement that the entire ligament becomes involved under stress. Amazingly enough, the anterior cruciate ligament may elongate up to 4 or 5 times its normal length under these laboratory conditions before actual disruption at one area occurs. As a result, when you are repairing cruciate injuries where the damage may be to various areas, it becomes difficult just to suture the visible point of rupture and hope that the entire ligament will survive. If you measure the anteromedial and posterolateral components, you see the extreme length of the ligament before the final rupture occurs. Under the miscroscope you can also observe multiple small ruptures occurring throughout the ligament.

As I mentioned we studied the anterior cruciate, the posterior cruciate, and the tibiocollateral ligament. There is quite a variation in the scanning structure of these ligaments; the anterior cruciate has rather wavy bundles with quite a lot of mucopolysaccarides in between the collagen fibrils, whereas the tibiocollateral ligament is much denser in its structure.

We examine these ligaments under four situations: (1) the relaxed normal ligament, (2) ligaments which our instron had subjected to minimal tension, (3) ligaments which had gone on to what the machine interpreted as failure, and (4) finally the total disruption that we can visibly see. The ligaments subjected to minimal tension have quite normal collagen fibrils; nothing really startling has occured under the scanning microscope. The main feature on the next group, which according to the instron had failed, is that with more tension the ligaments are not visibly disrupted but yet do not yield any resistance to the instron. When we removed these specimens and studied them under the scanning microscope, there were tremendous disruption of the collagen fibular architecture. Actually the microscopic pictures of the ligaments tested just to the point of visible disruption and of those that went on to total and entire failure were very similar. These findings suggest that when failure has been reached in tensile testing of ligaments, there is considerable disorganisation of the collagen arrangement throughout the substance of a ligament even though it still appears visibly intact.

Importance of Tests for Clinical Practice

The immediate clinical question of whether such collagen fibrils without visible disruption can with surgery reorientate, heal, and go on to perform normally is unfortunately a matter for speculation at this time. The concept of failure of a ligament which is visibly intact poses diagnostic and therapeutic problems. Antero-posterior instability in the presence of an intact ligament is clinically well known. Some of these ligaments may have been rendered function less with very little ability to resist any stress. The findings in this study demonstrate that ligaments may be stressed to all but failure in the absence of visible, macroscopic disruption.

3. Biomechanic Discussion of the Polyflex Ligament

M. E. Blazina

Prosthetic ligaments being investigated presently in the United States are the Polyflex ligament and the Proplast ligament. The principal investigators for the latter are Dr. SLOCUM and Dr. JAMES in Eugene, Oregon; Dr. HUGHSTON in Columbus, Georgia; and Dr. TULLOS and his group in Houston, Texas. The clinical and biomechanic properties of the Proplast ligament were recently discussed at the Annual Meeting of the American Academy of Orthopedic Surgeons in Las Vegas, Nevada, in February 1977. We would suggest that if anyone is interested in the Proplast ligament, he direct his questions toward Dr. JAMES. It was our impression upon hearing the presentation that the Proplast ligament was being modified again, and perhaps there will be alterations in the basic biomechanic data and in future clinical experiences.

Table 1. Richards Polyethylene Ligament Implant

Description

Hercules 1900 medical grade ultrahigh molecular weight polyethylene

6.35 mm in diameter

78 mm long after completed implantation

Reduced center section, 4.76 mm diameter and 35-40 mm length, represents the intra-articular ligament portions

Remaining, threaded length represents the extra-articular (or intraosseous) ligament portions. Each end of the implant is formed into a 0.25 × 20 mm lateral, having been cut to this length with a small bone cutter after implantation

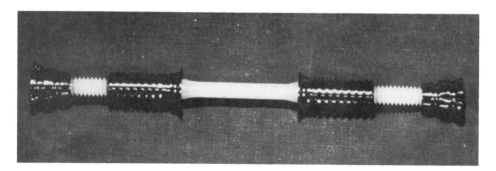

Fig. 1

Properties of Richards Polyflex Ligament

Properties of the Richards Polyflex ligament are listed in Table 1 and Figure 1 shows a photograph of the synthetic ligament. The Polyflex ligament is made of essentially the same material now being used both as the cup segment of total high replacement and the usual tibial plateau components of knee replacements.

Results of Laboratory Testing

Tables 2-4 contain data accumulated by testing the Polyflex ligament and comparing its performance with cadaver cruciate ligaments. Most of the information provided here comes from the work of Dr. NOYES, which has been published in the American volumes of the Journal of Bone and Joint Surgery. Some of the other information is derived from testing performed by the Richards Manufacturing Company. Dr. KENNEDY already has alluded to the fact that in vitro testing of a knee ligament may not represent a true in vivo situation. It is important to realize that one is not questioning the specific data itself, but rather its real meaning in relationship to the dynamics of the actual knee. Also, we would like to point out that there have been certain technical problems in the in vivo testing situations. Be that as it may, the information accumulated thus far has been and is being utilized to set the parameters for a standard cruciate ligament performance.

The first test (see Table 2) is the residual elongation test. A force of 230 N (newtons) elongated the Polyflex ligament 0.45 mm. This represents a force approximately of 60 lb, or 27 kg. Therefore at an elongating force of about 25 kg, one can elongate the Polyflex ligament and it will stay residually elongated. Incidentally, this force described by Dr. NOYES as being capable of residually elongating the Polyflex ligament is smaller than that described by Dr. KENNEDY. On the other hand, the normal anterior cruciate ligament will withstand greater residual elongation forces, as will shortly be discussed. If one reduces the elongation force to 117 N (~ 30 lb or 14 kg), there remains only a small unmeasurable residual elongation after the test. At an elongation force of 273 N (71 lb or 32 kg), full recovery was not achieved.

Dr. NOYES has stated that the anterior cruciate ligament in the younger adult human will withstand an elongation force of 200-400 N (i.e., 50-100 lb or 25-50 kg). Also, Dr. NOYES feels that the anterior cruciate ligament in older patients is weaker. Here again, he is trying to point out that the human anterior cruciate ligament is stronger than the Polyflex ligament. There is one important point in the residual elongation test that we would wish to reemphasize, which Dr. KENNEDY pointed out. Dr. NOYES does not take into account those probably lesser forces in clinical situations that do not disrupt the ligament, but do indeed render it nonfunctional. Besides the clinical situations described by Dr. KENNEDY, we would like to recall another rather familiar phenomenon. When fractured femurs were being treated extensively in skeletal traction, it was known that 20-25 lb really represented the maximum amount of traction we would like to apply steadily. In some cases where 50 lb or more had been applied for more than 24 hours, some damage to the cruciate ligaments occurred. In

Table 2. Richards Polyethylene Ligament Implant

_____

Tensile Tests

A. Residual elongation tests: single load-unload cycles in tension at increasing increments of force.

Force of 230 N: elongated to 0.45 mm; viscoelastic recovery after 1 s with residual elongation of 0.15%

Force of 117 N: small unmeasurable residual elongation exists 1 s after test

Force of 273 N: full recovery not achieved after 90 min

In vivo forces applied to anterior cruciate ligament range 200-400 N (younger adult humans) and 80-160 N (older adult humans)

For posterior cruciate ligament: force levels increase

Older human adults: force of 294 N required to elongate 10%

B. Cyclic creep tests

1. Measured during 1 cps tensile load-unload cycles to determine long term creep properties

100 cycles: elongates 1 mm

1010 cycles: elongates 2 mm

250,000 cycles: elongates 7.6 mm; after 1000 s shortened 3.1 mm

2. Measured at varying loading

20 lb: creep stops after 1 week
25 lb: creep stops after 3 weeks
30 lb: still occurring (at reduced rate) after 4 weeks

C. Fatigue tests: number of flexural (bending) cycles necessary for fatigue failure of ligament

Bending while immersed in 0.9 N saline at 37° C

After 81 million cycles: 10% reduction in stiffness and marked reduction in ductility

Failure occurred through section of reduced diameter at a stress of 25 megapascals and on elongation of 110%. (Normal implant failed at a stress of 40 megapascals at nearly 350% elongation)

After 3 million cycles no change in mechanical properties observed

_____

fact, X-rays taken with 50 lb of traction applied sometimes showed distraction of the knee joint. If one can already get into trouble with cruciate ligaments by applying forces less than those described by Dr. NOYES, then the apparent gap between human cruciate ligament performance and Polyflex ligament performance in the residual elongation test becomes somewhat smaller. On the other hand, we would wish to point out our concern about this apparent deficiency in the residual elongation test performance of the Polyflex ligament, and have always suggested that maximum stresses should be avoided, especially those that may arise in trying to return to competitive athletics.

The cyclic creep test, also shown in Table 2, is a modification of the residual elongation test. After loading and unloading repetitively, one then observes how long the tested ligament creeps. As can be noted, after 100 loading-unloading cycles the ligament elongated 1 mm. The other, somewhat different test seems to indicate once again that for the Polyflex ligament the critical range lies between 20-25 lb of loading.

Fatigue tests represent bending cycles, also shown in Table 2. Dr. NOYES and the Richards Manufacturing Company have both built machines that bend the knee rhythmically all day long, day after day. Dr. NOYES showed that after 81,000,000 cycles there was a 10% reduction in stiffness and a marked reduction in ductility. This observation is probably beyond the limit of human endurance. You would have to live a very long time and do a lot of jogging. On the other hand, after 3,000,000 cycles no change in the mechanical properties of the Polyflex ligament was noted. As an observation, therefore, performance of the Polyflex ligament in the fatigue test was apparently satisfactory.

A critical test for the Polyflex ligament has been the torsion test, as shown in Table 3. The Polyflex ligament fails with forces that are not very strong. This means that in its present configuration and constituency the Polyflex ligament will not tolerate rotational stresses of a significant degree. As has been pointed out elsewhere at this meeting, initially, at the time of the introduction of the Polyflex ligament, we were not aware of the effect of the rotational instabilities, particularly anterolateral instability in instances of anterior instability, and posterolateral instability in instances of posterior instability. If these stresses are not obviated by juxta-articular autogenous procedures, the Polyflex ligament will fail. Incidentally, there is some conjecture about the possibility that a normal human anterior cruciate ligament will go on to failure if forced to try and withstand considerable repetitive rotational stresses.

Table 3. Richards Polyethylene Ligament Implant

Torque Test: torque necessary to twist the ligament and to determine the No. of revolutions necessary for failure

Four trials at 15 rad/min:

A. Torque after 2II rad: 3.5-4 in.-lb

B. Maximum Torque: 5 in.-lb

C. Revolutions to failure: 11-14 revolutions

D. Mode of failure: ligament knots up, fails in tension

E. Shear nodules (G) = 1.24×10^3 psi

Clinical Experience and Suggestions for Improvement

In reviewing the presented biomechanic data, one sees that there appear to be at least three areas of discussion for future improvement: fixation of the ligament, the composition of the ligament, and lastly, the configurative design of the ligament. The present ligament never was felt to represent an ultimate form of development. All knowledge is evolutionary and all technology eventuates in modification and improvement. That has been and always will be the story of engineering progress.

26

We would very much like to see some change in the method of fixation.
If we could have fibrous tissue ingrowth with a significant increase
in holding properties, that would certainly be welcomed in prosthetic
ligament replacement and, incidentally, in all types of joint replacement. Proplast purportedly has this property. Perhaps there are other
materials that will do likewise and should be investigated.

In regard to the composition of the ligament itself, it has always
been felt from the knowledge derived on a theoretical design basis
that the polyethylene probably needs to be impregnated with some
other material, possibly carbon, to improve its basic strength and to
increase its capability of withstanding elongation and cyclic phenomena. That modification represents an engineering problem. We hope that
work will be allowed to continue in this direction and progress be
made.

In regard to the configurative design of the ligament, it would appear
that the prosthetic cruciate ligament should be made up of numerous
fibrils in a woven fashion so as to be able to withstand rotational
stresses. Again, this represents an engineering problem, and we would
hope that something resembling the anatomic design of the human cruciate could eventually be developed.

Insofar as the sleeves are concerned, they would appear at the present
time to be essential in preventing erosion of the ligament at the
exit holes in the intercondylar region. The use of nuts would be
utilized only for temporary fixation if we could obtain eventual fibrous tissue ingrowth in the intraosseous regions.

In reviewing our clinical experience, we should like to point out
certain phenomena noted on follow-up examination. A postoperative
X-ray will show the nuts and sleeves (see Fig. 2). It also gives
some idea of the disposition of the methyl-methacrylate cement. One
cannot visualize the Polyflex ligament itself, as it is radiolucent;
however, one can get an idea about the placement and course of the
Polyflex ligaments. One case illustrated shows a loosened nut. Originally, loosening of the nut was attributed to too early mobilization,
although we have noted loosening even after immobilization. If nut
loosening represents an isolated phenomenon, the nut can be replaced
and refixated with methylmethacrylate cement.

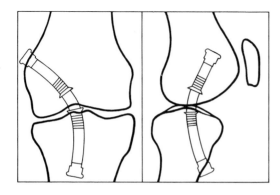

Fig. 2

Insofar as the sleeves are concerned, they can also loosen, which can sometimes be noted on X-ray. Other times it can only be visualized at arthroscopy or arthrotomy. Correction of a loosened sleeve causing significant symptoms would hecessitate taking down the entire ligament.

A broken ligament can occur for a variety of reasons. Site of insertion may cause condylar impingment and erosion of the ligament. Excoriation of a sleeve due to its being handled with metal tipped instruments may lead to ligament erosion. As described above, if significant rotational stresses exist residually, the ligament will probably fail, and perhaps in a short period of time. Also, the functional stresses applied on the knee may have exceeded the biomechanic properties of the ligament. For various reasons we have explored certain cases which have had a prosthetic cruciate ligament inserted 2 to 3 years later and found the ligament to be intact. Based on some of the above biomechanic observations, it is difficult to ascertain why these ligaments are still intact. Pertinent to this comment, one can look at Morrison's data, listed in Table 4. Some of the forces he describes are considerable, even for the normal human cruciate ligament. The cruciate ligaments in vivo certainly must be utilzing backup support.

Table 4. Morrison's in Vivo Measurements of the Cruciate Ligaments

	Anterior C.L. (N)	Posterior C.L. (N)
Level walking	169	352
Ascending stairs	67	641
Descending stairs	445	262
Ascending 9.45° ramp	27	1215
Descending 9.45° ramp	93	449

Discussion

COTTA: According to our experience, 3 hours after death there is a change of the ground substance, at which time alterations take place in the collagen structure and cells die. The elasticity is certainly also reduced during this process. What significance would you attribute to these facts, especially regarding synthetic material?

KENNEDY: During our initial experiments, the difficulty of immediately getting ligaments on an instron machine led us to store our ligaments in saline, sometimes for a period of 2, 3, or 4 days. The regardings were not as conclusive and definite as the readings which we had when we removed the ligaments and tested them within 3 or 4 hours after death. On the other hand, although I know you cannot relate humans to dogs, we have done dog experiments while trying to test synthetic ligaments. During these experiments we removed knee cruciates in the opposite knee almost at the time of death and tested them. We found that the ratio was about the same as in the cadaver.

The other aspect of our work which did not support NOYES is that surprisingly enough we did not really find much difference between the ligament strengths of younger individuals and older patients. One would naturally expect deterioration in strength, but some of our young patients in motor vehicle accidents exhibited cruciates which were not all that much stronger than those of older individuals.

KRAHL: I should like to enlarge on Dr. KENNEDY's comments. In Finland there is the group VIIDIK which has been concerned with the extent to which the postmortal structure of connective tissue can be compared with living tissue in regard to loading capacity. VIIDIK found out that directly after death structural changes can be seen both with the electron microscope and the light microscope, but that the biomechanic parameter does not change in a period of 92 hours if the milieu of the ligament or tendon is maintained, e.g., at a temperature of 22° in a tyrode solution.

BRUSSATIS: I would be interested in asking Dr. BLAZINA a few questions about the bone structure at the special points where the ligaments are anchored. I am referring to the distribution of the loading forces on the two points above and below the anchoring of the ligaments. Some investigations have been done concerning the special architecture of the bone, especially cancellous bone. Is there any microscopic destruction, and are there reasons for distributing the loading forces in another manner? I would think there would be some very critical weakening of the bone structures at that point.

BLAZINA: We would agree; as I mentioned, one of the problems is fixation, not only intraosseous fixation, but also that of the stresses placed on methylmethacrylate bone interface. That is one of the toughest We would prefer dealing with compression force or some other rather than a sheer force. On the other hand, this is all that we have today. Obviously the ultimate type of fixation will be incorporation of the ligament into the bone. That will have to come, and I think that it will come. This is a very critical point. Incidental, testing this ligament in a cadaver with methylmethacrylate is useless.

I would like to make a point, and it is that whether we are talking about athletes or about people involved in repetitive activity in general, when the tendons do rupture, you may not have had a normal tendon. Damage can occur at a very early age, depending upon the stresses that have been applied to these tendons or ligaments. This is a point that again is very difficult to demonstrate in the laboratory.

O'DONOGHUE: Dr. KENNEDY, would you enlarge on your comment in regard to what happens to the ligament which is stressed to less than its ultimate destruction. In other words, it seems to me that some experiments would be in order to determine what happened to this ligament if it were maximally and heavily stressed. I think this is a very valuable clinical contribution, because admittedly, if I check a ligament which has been stressed and which seems intact but whose substance is in fact not intact, then it is of great interest whether this ligament of the knee will ever return to normal strength and length or whether it will always be inadequate. Can you comment?

KENNEDY: We thought about the clinical aspects of this problem a lot, but they are difficult to reduplicate in an experiment. We cannot do it in humans because we would have to deal with cadaver material. We thought about doing it in dogs, but is is hard to stress an anterior cruciate ligament in a live dog, then take out a specimen, determine that it has not gone to ultimate, visible disruption, but just to a point of microscopic failure, then close the knee joint and simply hope that the remaining fibers showing microscopic disruption will recover or not recover to a normal condition. I do not believe we can do this in an experiment.

BLAZINA: In a review of our records of patients with posterior instability of the knee, we determined that for about half the patients, the previous surgeon had said the anterior cruciate ligament was intact. The surgeon stated in these recods that the posterior cruciate ligament was torn, that he repaired it, and that the anterior cruciate ligament looked fine. These cases failed and went on to further surgery. In most of these cases, when the surgeons went in the second time, they discovered that the anterior cruciate ligament was gone.

In conclusion, I feel that we need not only a laboratory evaluation of this phenomenon but also a clinical evaluation of the statics of inquired ligaments, especially of the anterior cruciate ligament at the time of initial surgery.

KRAHL: If I understood Dr. KENNEDY correctly, he said that he interpreted the influence of the speed of deformation in his elasticity investigations such that a higher speed of deformation leads to a stiffening of the ligaments, which implies a greater elasticity at lower speed of deformation. We were able to achieve similar results in our investigations on patella tendons and foot tendons. It is interesting that at a speed of approximately 10 m/sec, loading rates were found which were 50% higher than at a speed 10 times lower. Furthermore, we were able to recognize the influence of age and sex. Can you confirm these results?

KENNEDY: It was not quite clear; you still said that at very rapid loading rates the ligaments resisted more? I think we could confirm that.

HOHMANN: Dr. BLAZINA, you showed us a lot of fatigue tests of polyethylene. Do you have results on the behavior of polyethylene in the human body over a long period of time, including the aging of the material and the changing of material properties over the years?

BLAZINA: We routinely perform synovial biopsy. If we have some reason to do arthroscopy postsurgery, we also do a synovial biopsy. There is a point up to which the knee can tolerate some of the degenerative changes occurring with the polyethylene. One can find a subclinical synovial reaction. On the other hand, there is a point at which problems with the replacement are such that the knee will not tolerate it. These cases will have chronic synovitis with chronic effusion, and the foreign-body reaction will be much greater. This is not to be confused with an infection. There is a reaction, and one can detect it in the synovium. On the other hand, there are some cases where the synovium is perfectly normal.

HOHMANN: I think my question was about change in the polyethylene itself over a period of time; I mean changing of material properties and n ot reaction of the joint or tissue.

BLAZINA: Yes, there is change; however, when one analyzes failures of the ligament, one must first rule out technique and combinations of instability which may not have been treated originally. On the other hand we don't know a lot about the long-term changes. Some intact ligaments which for other reasons had to be taken out showed no structural change after 1 or 2 years. The question as to long-term changes is a good one but presently impossible to answer.

O'DONOGHUE: Dr. KENNEDY, did you ever put the polyethylene material under the electron microscope?

KENNEDY: Like in all operations, we had some failures and some good results with the high-density polyethylene. In the case of failure and breakage, which we experienced several times after earlier operations, we usually did look at them under the scanning microscope. There were some surface imperfections in the polyethylene which eventually led to cleavage, erosion and breakage. In those cases, we thought that it was not so much the nature of the material as it was the method by which the ligament initially was manufactured that caused the problem. Many of these breaks had a lot of surface fissuring on them, and I don't think it was because of our technique and implantation at that time.

MOSCHI: We have been working on the biomechanics of the anterior cruciate. Our problem does not deal as much with the tensile properties and failure of the anterior cruciate as with its plastic module. The point at which the collagen fibrils start to fail is the same point at which the plastic module registers failure as well. It is here that we also see most of our failures at surgery. The problem is this: We know that the module of elongation of collagen is about 5% of that of a tendon. When we test the anterior cruciate ligament, we have a module of elongation of about 60% before we see tears in the fibers with the scanning electron microscope. But if we test the ligamentum flavum, or a small, elastic artery by stressing it with the same elongation, the artery will not give way. That means that the connective tissue of the anterior cruciate and of the arteries supplying blood to the anterior cruciate do not break at the same elongation. If we have a tear of the anterior cruciate ligament and a tear in the plastic module, we still think that the blood supply is there just because we know that the little arteries with their larger elastic supply will not break until after the collagen fibrils.

Do you think it proper to repair a ligament in a situation like this? If you leave the ligament as it is, you have the opportunity to have a blood supply and then to revascularize the ligament. On the other hand, you cannot be certain whether the ligament is going to be longer or return to normal length. If you do decide to put stitches in this ligament, you close what probably remained of the blood supply. The dilemma is that in this case you can really go more in the opposite direction, namely that for a short time you are going to have a mechanical ligament that is shorter but without a blood supply. I would like to have your opinion on this subject and possibly also that of Dr. TRILLAT, who I know is very interested in this problem.

KENNEDY: That is a very interesting observation. The saying cropped up in Memphis, Tennessee, 2 or 3 weeks ago that spaghetti was for eating and not sewing. I guess that applies here, but to answer your question, having followed a series of 50 cases of tears of the anterior cruciate ligament where we either repaired the ligaments or did not repair them, just ignoring them-particularly the midcruciate - we determined at the end of 44 months that 80% of the patients ended up in good or excellent condition, regardless of treatment. We carried that follow-up to 88 months and found that the failure quota in patients with severe complications rose to 35%. Therefore, my answer to your question would be that if you believe you can do something to make the anterior cruciate ligament survive, by all means do it.

TRILLAT: The posterior cruciate ligament is supplied from arteries with small volumes of blood simultaneously in its upper, central, and lower parts. This is why its vitality is often prolonged even in the case of either an old or new traumatic rupture. Therefore, even late reconstruction is possible.

In contrast, the anterior cruciate ligament is poorly vascularized. It only receives blood from one small artery in the upper part, and it is therefore probable that its blood supply has to come partly from the bony areas where it is fixed and partly from the synovial envelope surrounding it. This explains why it is often the case that in an old instability no trace of the anterior cruciate ligament can be found. This also explains that the rupture can occur in the interior of the synovial sheath. The latter can become enlarged following a trauma, due to increased circulation. This explains that when trauma occurs, if the anterior cruciate ligament is already functionally deficient, then only the synovium is ruptured, which leads to the syndrome of repeated hemarthrosis. This syndrome is the best way of confirming both that the anterior cruciate has been torn in the initial accident and that the synovium which covers it is not only intact but also enlarged and slightly bleeding.

We must add that in this enlarged synovial tube, the anterior cruciate may tend towards the posterior cruciate, attach itself to it, and be nourished by it. It is therefore easy surgically to separate the two and to reinsert the nonatrophic anterior cruciate in the upper part, which has been well nourished in the period following the trauma.

WEBER: As far as I have understood, vascularization is of great importance in the healing process of the anterior cruciate ligament. However, I do not understand how a ligament, reconstructed out of fascia and tendon, is nourished when there is not a single vessel in it. There is no intermedial vessel, no synovial vessel. Could you explain how long revascularization takes and whether there is a revascularization or not?

TRILLAT: This is a question of great importance, which I can answer with two considerations.

I had to reoperate only one of my own patients to remove a small, irritating foreign body. Three years previously, I had preformed a reconstruction of the anterior cruciate according to the Kenneth Jones method, modified by ERIKSSON. During the second operation I was able to confirm that the transplanted tendon was vital, surrounded by a neosynovium, and that the latter was larger than at the time of transplantation.

However, to be quite honest, I do not think that this is the usual development. If I continue to be so enthusiastic about the reconstruction of the anterior cruciate ligament as does ERIKSSON, then it is for the following reasons:

In the majority of cases, surgical intervention in acute or chronic instabilities does not only mean in my opinion the reconstruction of the central pivot, but also of the peripheral ligaments. Peripheral reconstruction alone, at least in the initial period, does not restore to the knee a perfect recentralization of the joint; with the slightest flexion or rotation, the abnormal tensions effect the area which is healing. This, little by little, leads to a new distension and therefore to a chronic instability and to failure.

However, if a suture of the anterior cruciate is carried out, for a certain length of time everything will be as if it were a normal knee. The healing of the peripheral elements would therefore be satisfactory.

If there is also atrophy of the central reconstructed ligament, the knee is then like a normal knee on which a simple cut of the anterior cruciate ligament has been carried out. We know that in this case no problem occurs and in particular that there is no indication of an anterior drawer sign.

These are the two reasons which always lead me to reconstruct the central pivot (column).

4. Classification of Knee Joint Instability Resulting From Ligamentous Damage

J. C. Kennedy

At present, our working classification for knee joint instability is
confusing, but we are struggling to clarify its terminology by pooling
resources from major knee centers throughout North America just as
was done a decade ago with scoliosis. In the past, dislocations of the
knee were simply but perhaps incorrectly classified as medial, lateral,
posterior, anterior, and rotatory on the basis of the direction in which
the tibia was displaced. Although useful, the classification represented
over-simplification, avoiding three-plane instabilities which commonly
occur with disrupted knees.

This classification attempts to describe the instability by the direction of the tibial displacement and, if possible, by structural
deficits. It refers to instability occurring from acute trauma or from
acute instability progressing to a chronic state, ignoring congenital
and acquired instability from other causes. (i.e., tibial plateau
fractures, congenital hyperextension, etc.)

Classification

Our working classification for knee joint instability resulting from
ligamentous damage includes the following:

A. One-plane instabilities
   1. One-plane medial
   2. One-plane lateral
   3. One-plane posterior
   4. One-plane anterior

B. Rotatory instabilities
   1. Anteromedial
   2. Anterolateral
      In flexion
      Approaching extension
   3. Posterolateral
   4. Posteromedial

C. Combined instabilities
   1. Anterolateral-posterolateral rotatory
   2. Anterolateral-anteromedial rotatory
   3. Anteromedial-posteromedial rotatory

Discussion

This is an anatomic classification, i.e., one-plane medial instability means the tibia is moving away from the femur on the medial side. Anteromedial rotatory instability indicates that the tibia rotates anteriorly and moves away from the femur on the medial side.

The problem becomes more complex as attempts are made to include structural deficits. This is quite understandable. Individual surgeons encounter different pathological lesions which unfortunately stand out in their minds as the lesion producing a specific instability. In addition, biomechanic interpretation of cadaveric dissections often differ from accurate clinical and operative observations. Equally important is the realization that acute and chronic lesions of a structure may not follow identical pathological patterns about the knee joint.

Description of Classification

A. One-Plane Instabilities

1. One-Plane Medial Instability

Tested with the knee in complete extension. A valgus opening with the knee in complete extension represents one plane medial instability. The knee opens on the medial side, the tibia moving away from the femur. This represents a major instability. There is involvement of the tibial collateral ligament, the medial capsular ligament, the anterior cruciate ligament, the posterior oblique ligament, and the medial portion of the posterior capsule. It strongly suggests involvement of the posterior cruciate ligament but does not totally indite this structure.

Tested with the knee in 30° of flexion. There are a group of patients where the tibia moves away from the femur in flexion without appreciable clinical rotatory elements (i.e., grad I or grade II knee sprains). This depends on the severity of the involvement of medial structures.

2. One-Plane Lateral Instability

Tested with the knee in extension. The knee opens on the lateral side, the tibia moving away from the femur. Structures involved include the lateral capsular ligament, fibular collateral ligament, biceps tendon either partial or complete, arcuate-popliteus complex (partial or complete), the anterior cruciate ligament, and commonly the posterior cruciate ligament. This is a major instability, approaching the proportions of a dislocation.

Tested with the knee in 30° of flexion. One should again be cognisant that minor one-plane lateral instability may be present in 30° of flexion without major pathology.

3. One-Plane Posterior Instability

In this situation, the tibia is displaced posteriorly with the knee in a semi-flexed position (i.e., automobile dashboard injury or direct blow on the tibial crest). The structures involved include the posterior arcuate ligament, arcuate ligament complex (partial or complete), and posterior oblique ligament complex (partial or complete). Whereas initially the damage may seem confined solely to the posterior cruciate ligament, chronic one-plane posterior instability eventually may involve the posteromedial and posterolateral corners, such areas demanding close evaluation and consideration for reinforcement when dealing with this instability.

4. One-Plane Anterior Instability

Because of diverse theories currently in vogue, this disability is difficult to comprehend fully. The tibia in neutral position moves forward on the femur. Structures involved naturally include the anterior cruciate ligament, the lateral capsular ligament (partial or complete), and medial capsular ligament (partial or complete). The anterior drawer sign is positive in neutral position if the anterior cruciate ligament is involved with immediate or subsequent stretching of the medial and lateral capsules. Although laboratory studies suggest involvement of only a portion of the anterior cruciate ligament in producing an anterior drawer sign, the injury clinically suggests loss of functional integrity of the entire ligament.

B. Rotatory Instabilities

1. Anteromedial Rotatory Instability

In this situation, the medial plateau of the tibia rotates anteriorly with the joint opening on the medial side. Structures involved include the medial capsular ligament, tibial collateral ligament, posterior oblique ligament, and anterior cruciate ligament. This instability seems best understood. The researcher merely has to cut these structures in sequence in the cadaver to see the sequential and orderly progression of anteromedial rotatory instability.

2. Anterolateral Rotatory Instability

A. In flexion. This instability has really little to do with major anterior displacement of the tibia. The lateral tibial plateau rotates forward in relationship to the femur at 90° with excessive lateral opening (a tendency for excessive internal rotation of the tibia on the femur with the knee in flexion). Structures involved include the lateral capsular ligament, arcuate ligament complex (partial), and anterior cruciate ligament (partial or complete).

B. Approaching extension (anterior subluxation of the lateral tibial plateau. With a specific test, the lateral tibial plateau subluxates forward on the femur as the knee approaches extension. Structures involved include the anterior cruciate ligament and possible involvement of the lateral capsular ligament. With the knee coming into extension, one has the dramatic anterior subluxation of the lateral tibial plateau as the weight-bearing extremity begins to extend.

3. Posterolateral Rotatory Instability

The lateral tibial plateau rotates posteriorly in relationship to the femur with lateral opening. Structures involved include the arcuate ligament complex, biceps tendon, anterior cruciate ligament (partial or complete), lateral capsular ligament, and at times stretching or loss of integrity of the posterior cruciate ligament. It is important to distinguish this type of instability from one-plane posterior instability resulting from a tear of the posterior cruciate ligament. In the disability under discussion, the posterolateral corner of the tibia drops off the back of the femur and there is a varus opening.

4. Posteromedial Rotatory Instability

In this situation, the medial tibial plateau rotates posteriorly in reference to the femur with medial opening. Structures involved include the tibial collateral ligament, medial capsular ligament, posterior oblique ligament, anterior cruciate ligament, the medial portion of the posterior capsule, and stretching or major involvement of the semimembranosus system. A hyperextension valgus force can tear these structures, the anterior cruciate ligament tearing before the posterior cruciate ligament, which is only mildly stretched. The resulting instability is a sagging back of the posteromedial corner of the tibia on the femur with valgus opening.

C. Combined Instabilities

One-plane and rotatory instabilities are soon understood. Structural deficits are mildly debatable with such instabilities. However, combined instabilities compound this problem. Each orthopedic surgeon will have to satisfy his own beliefs as to what structures are specifically damaged and their relative degree of involvement in combined instabilities.

1. Combined Anterolateral-Posterolateral Rotatory Instability

In this situation the lateral tibial plateau rotates in a posterior direction. But when additionally tested, exhibits excessive forward displacement of the lateral tibial plateau on the femur. Naturally, the lateral instability is great with excessive damage to the majority of structures on the lateral side of the knee.

2. Combined Anterolateral-Anteromedial Rotatory Instability

This is a common instability. The major posterior structures are spared. The examiner may demonstrate excessive anterior rotation of the medial tibial plateau (that is, abnormal external rotatory instability). In addition, the examiner can readily produce positive anterior subluxation of the lateral tibial plateau as the knee approaches extension.

3. Combined Anteromedial-Posteromedial Rotatory Instability

In this situation, medial and posteromedial structures are severely involved. The knee opens on the medial side, the tibia moving away from the femur. The tibia may rotate anteriorly when tested, but, in addition, with further testing the tibia moves in the opposite direction, rotating posteriorly and dropping off the posteromedial corner.

All medial structures including the semimembranosus complex are involved in combination with the anterior and most likely with the posterior cruciate ligaments.

4. *Further Combined Instabilities*

An outline of further combined instabilities which would include
three-plane or even six-plane dimensions would be both confusing
and impractical. The variation in structural deficits would create
major confusion. Using the above classification, the orthopedic
surgeon should again an insight and understanding of the more complex
instabilities.

Discussion

SCHULITZ: Do you agree with Professor HUGHSTON's argument against the
existence of a posteromedial rotatory instability?

KENNEDY: No! We intend to change his mind in one month's time. We have
had many discussions about this, and actually, I think I have convinced
him. He feels that it doesn't exist because he feels you cannot internally rotate the tibia on the femur without disruption of the end of
the posterior cruciate ligament. If you have disruption, then it becomes a dislocated knee. However, in our input from 20 centers in the
United States there were many people who saw that instability with an
intact posterior cruciate ligament.

SCHULITZ: What is your opinion, Dr. O'DONOGUE?

O'DONOGUE: I agree with what Dr. KENNEDY just said. I think you can
have a posteromedial rotatory instability with an intact posterior
cruciate ligament. I would vote with Dr. KENNEDY against Dr. HUGHSTON;
I have operated with the purpose of reconstructing the posterior cruciate ligament for posteromedial instability, only to find that it
was intact.

SCHULITZ: Dr. MOSCHI, can you as a former assistant of Professor
HUGHSTON agree with this?

MOSCHI: First of all, I do not agree with Dr. BLAZINA because I believe
there is no such thing as an acute posteromedial rotatory instability.
This is probably one of the cases requiring a division into chronic
and acute instability. We are speaking now of a classification that
is just anatomic and not biomechanic. If you employ a biomechanic
classification such as that of the school of Professor TRILLAT, then
such a thing as posteromedial rotatory instability becomes conceivable.

Secondly, how do you check a posteromedial rotatory instability? We
have two signs to prove it. The first is the drawer with the tibia
internally rotated. When we try to check the second Slocum sign, we
must be sure that we perform this test with the same internal rotation that we have in the opposite, normal knee, i.e., if in the
opposite, normal knee we have an internal rotation of about 15°, we
must likewise have the affected knee in 15° of internal rotation, but
not in 30°. Otherwise we will not be testing the posterior cruciate
anymore, but instead something else, namely the lateral capsule. As-
suming you have an intact posterior cruciate and you perform such an
internal rotation as for the drawer test, if the knee wants to slide
posteromedially, it must change the center of rotation. Since we
are adhering to an anatomic and not a biomechanic classification, it
is practicably impossible with a knee that has only tears in the
posteromedial corner to perform a physiological internal rotation
without tying up the posterior cruciate. When you tie up the posterior
cruciate you go to a locked position called a close-packed position, and

in this position you can no longer test any kind of instability. Obviously this is just an opinion, based on our clinical observations of acute tears of the medial compartment of quite varying sizes. If you do not have a tear of the posterior cruciate, you will never have a drop back in the medial compartment.

SCHULITZ: Are you convinced, Dr. BLAZINA?

BLAZINA: I think that we should spend a lot more time on the classification rather than go into the argumentation. One thing that I don't like about this classification right off the bat is that you are ignoring the valgus and varus instability as a major form of classification. In reconstruction there is a point in which varus or valgus instability may occur. If you tighten these instabilities anteromedially, anterolaterally, posterolaterally, and posteromedially but do not tighten them in varus or valgus, you lose the game. I do not see how you can have a workable classification without varus and valgus in there.

KENNEDY: We did not have one-plane medial or one-plane lateral; that is varus and valgus.

BLAZINA: I thought that was a theoretical classification.

KENNEDY: We argued about this and I think the answer is an anatomic classification. If you believe that there is no such thing as posteromedial rotatory instability, then obviously you do not use it. The one situation where we have seen it is in a hyperextension valgus injury where the degree of hyperextension has torn the anterior cruciate and the posteromedial corner but has not torn the posterior cruciate ligament. We have acute knees where we have explored them and found this situation. We know it exists, yet if a group does not believe in it, then that's fine. We are not wearing any medals for this classification.

MOSCHI: We saw something like that when I was in Columbus, Georgia, with the Football Kickers. With a hyperextension there was a tear of the anterior cruciate of the medial compartment, but usually the posterior cruciate was a little loose in those cases. As a result, you could have posteromedial instability because of the looseness of the posterior cruciate. It should be demonstrated that this did not happen at the instant centers of rotation, but if we do that, we lose their anatomic classification and we got over to a biomechanic classification. It just depends on our hands and what we are going to do later.

KARPF: Dr. KENNEDY, is the distinction between a simple instability and a rotatory instability at all possible? I think the simple instabilities you mentioned are just a description of the accident mechanism. If you have a valgus instability and the entire medial capsule with the dorsal cup is ruptured, then it is no longer a simple instability, but a rotatory instability. I think that the definitions are overlapping; therefore, the table is perhaps not so good.

KENNEDY: I did not include in the table that we also feel that there is a one-plane valgus or varus instability with the knee in 30° of flexion; as Dr. JAMES pointed out, there also may be a degree of valgus without a major rotatory element. We have therefore included the simple skiing injury where the knee is flexioned to 30°, in which position it does open the valgus as part of a one-plane instability.

I think that this should be included, because it may make a difference in when you operate on such a patient.

HERTEL: Dr. KENNEDY, you know the experiments on cadaver knees done by WARREN, who found out that rotatory instability increased only when the upper layers of the medial collateral ligament were also damaged. No increased rotatory instability is present when only the deeper layers of the medial collateral ligament are severed and the upper layers are intact.

KENNEDY: All we can say is this: There is a reprint here in which we reported studies on cases of medial instability where we felt dividing in sequence the capsular ligament initially produced both an opening on the medial side and an element of external rotation or lateral rotation. As you then divide the capsular ligament and finally the anterior cruciate, all elements increased. However, there is other work that has been done where they feel that the capsule may remain reasonably intact, and you can tear a portion of the tibiocollateral ligament and get an valgus opening in the knee joint.

O'DONOGHUE: I think what is happening is the very thing that we were trying to prevent happening. We found it impossible to get any unanimity of opinion concerning classification until we knew what we meant by what we said. All this anatomic classification is only trying to describe what is happening, what is involved, and what instability is. It is trying to say that when you have anteromedial rotatory instability, there is always a certain combination of things involved; as you all know from having seen acute injuries, you may have various combinations of injuries and still have the same clinical instability. I think that the contribution that KENNEDY has been making is that we at least know what place we are starting from. From then on, of course, what you decide to do about it is debatable, as you can see from this discussion. I think that if you have one thing in mind which has been talked about for 25 years now, and that is, if you repair everything that is torn, then you probably have solved the problem, whatever the problem was.

5. Diagnosis of Different Instabilities

D. H. O'Donoghue

Goals of Treatment

In order to obtain a good clinical end result from treatment, we need to know our goals in diagnosis:

Accept athletics
Avoid expediency
Adopt best method of treatment
Act promptly
Achieve perfection

Accept athletics. Since most of the knee joints to be treated are in athletes, I think you need to believe in athletics. It needs to be important to the doctor that his patient be restored to whatever activity the patient wants to do, not to whatever the doctor wants him to do.

Avoid expediency. Too often outside influences may overbalance sound judgement. The player's desire to compete, one's own overoptimism, failure to admit the extent of the damage, or hesitation to interfere with school attendance may lead one to adopt a "middle of the road" course. Strict medical evaluation, not temporary convenience, must be the deciding factor.

Adopt the best method of treatment. Sometimes it is easier to put the patient in a cast than to operate him, or in an elastic bandage rather than a cast. However, you must steel yourself to do what is the best thing, not the easiest thing.

Act promptly. Once you do decide what is wrong with this young person and know what would be the best treatment for him, you ought to proceed with it. We have a great tendency to put a patient in a cast for a while when in doubt. This might be acceptable for a few days in order to let the pain and apprehension subside somewhat. But if you put him in a cast for 6 weeks, you have then decided that you are not going to do surgical treatment. If you are going to do surgical treatment, it must be done at once. You have to make up your mind, diagnose what is wrong with the patient, decide what would be the best thing to do for him, and then act.

Achieve perfection. Of course, this last goal may seem a bit ridiculous, but you will not achieve perfection if you do not try for it. You have to try to get the patient entirely well or you certainly shall not accomplish it.

Clinical Picture

Diagnosis is a pretty broad subject when all the knee ligaments are considered. Diagnosis of knee ligament injury demands early, meticulous and complete examination. Note particularly:

Apparent severity of injury
Restriction or pain on normal motion
Presence of abnormal motion
Location and extent of tenderness
Amount and rapidity of the swelling
Location of swelling - intra- or extrasynovial
Deformity, either present or reported
Locking, if present

In reconstruction, many times the examination cannot be early, but the sooner you get to work on the reconstruction, the better. You need to get the show on the road. In other words, you need to make up your mind what this patient needs as soon as you can.

As for the severity of the injury, there is sometimes a great difference between instability and disability. I think it is possible to have what would be interpreted as an unstable knee which does not bother at all. If this instability is not severe enough that it would cause later arthritic changes, I think this patient would not need a reconstruction. Those two terms are not necessarily synonymous.

Someone asked what I would do when operating a knee with an acute injury consisting of a torn meniscus and also a torn anterior cruciate ligament that could not be repaired. I would not reconstruct it at that point, but I would have to wait until the patient had obvious symptoms of instability. (I should have known that before I even operated him.) Many people can, I think, get along without their anterior cruciate ligament if the rest of the ligaments are tight. You will have a better, more cooperative patient (which is extremely important), if he has recognized the fact that he does have trouble rather than your having to persuade him that he will have trouble later on.

A general examination should be made for swelling, tenderness, and range of motion. This is pretty routine. I think you should make a habit of examining the opposite knee first. There are two reasons for this: (1) to give the patient an idea what you are going to do, and (2) you will get some idea of what this person's normal state probably is.

Clinical Aspects of Knee Anatomy

Although I will not spend a lot of time discussing anatomy, I think my concept of the knee needs a little explanation (Fig. 1). When we dissect the knee, we take out all those ligaments and end up with multiple little bands and tendons and little strips of ligament. That is well and good to know, but I think the most important things to consider are: (1) What are these ligaments for? (2) What do they do? (3) How do they act? My concept of the ligaments of the knee is that they are all one big correlated group. On extension of the knee, the femoral condyles settle back into a sleeve, or a cuff, or a pocket of ligaments. You can call them anything you want to, but the main thing is that this is a pretty solid cuff all the way around, from about the midline on the medial side in front, around the back side and extends to the midline laterally. What you want to do is restore that cuff, and the less dissection you do, the less stripping out you do, the better function you should get. You are not doing a dissection now. You are doing a reconstruction. It is very important that the nerve and blood supply be preserved. You may make a beautiful reconstruction, but if you sever the nerves, the reconstruction will not last very long.

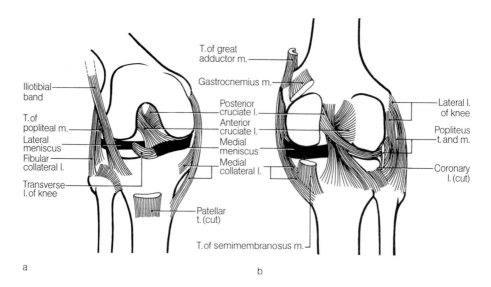

Fig. 1. Ligaments of the knee. a Anterior view. The patellar tendon is sectioned and the patella reflected upward. The knee is flexed at 90°. b Posterior view. Knee extended [1]

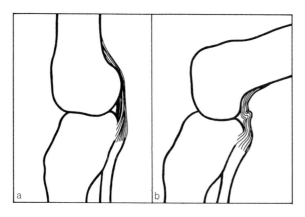

Fig. 2. Posterior capsule. a Tight with the knee in extension. b Redundant and no longer a stabilizer in flexion [1]

I would like to say a few words about the posterior capsule. I think the posterior capsule is extremely important in knee stability, but it has the handicap that once the knee is flexed a bit, it no longer functions as a stabilizer of the knee (Fig. 2). With the posterior capsule tight, you can take off either the medial or lateral ligaments and the knee will remain stable in adduction or abduction. However, if you flex the knee a little bit, then the posterior capsule no longer is functioning to stop either overextension or lateral motion. I will say a little more about this later.

This also applies to the anterior cruciate and the posterior cruciate. In a knee ligament injury you do need to know what has been injured. This is important for rehabilitation as well, because many times it may be difficult to decide whether there is medial or lateral instability in an old chronic knee. However, if you go back into the history and find out what happened to the patient, you will get a very valuable clue as to what he has. You can have instability with the biicomponents injured, which fits in with my suggestion that the ligaments together make a solid cuff rather than a bunch of avascular strips of tissue.

The medial side components include the long fibers of the medial collateral ligament, the medial capsular ligament, the medial meniscus, and the medial posterior capsule. The same is true on the lateral side of the knee. The posterior components consist of the posterior cruciate, the posterior capsule, plus all these oblique ligaments already demonstrated. The purpose of all these components is to form a solid cuff to stabilize the knee. It makes a lot of difference if there is more than one component that is injured. Also, if you have the posteromedial capsule and the medial collateral ligaments gone, you will probably have the anterior cruciate gone too. This is a much more serious injury than if you had any one of them alone. The anterior and the posterior cruciates have been studied pretty well. In our anxiety to get these cruciate ligaments involved in rotation and rotational instabilities, I think we sometimes forget that their primary function is to protect the anteroposterior stability.

Location of Injury

For the examination you want to end up knowing what combination is damaged and then be prepared to take care of that particular thing. In medial side injuries, all of the following structures may be damaged:

Medial collateral ligament
Anterior cruciate ligament
Medial meniscus
Posterior capsule
Posterior cruciate
Patellar retinaculum
Patellar tendon
Lateral meniscus

These may remain damaged when the patient comes in for his reconstruction operation.

We already discussed some of the lateral side injuries, which include:

Fibular collateral ligament
Iliotibial band
Lateral meniscus
Posterior cruciate ligament
Posterior capsule
Anterior cruciate ligament
Biceps tendon
Peroneal nerve
Popliteus tendon
Medial meniscus

In this complex injury, the peroneal nerve can be damaged; it is probably one of the most important structures to identify and to recognize in whatever procedure you are going to do on the lateral side of the knee. Before you operate, it is very important to know the status of the peroneal nerve; there may be some damage remaining from the original injury which, if unrecognized before surgery, may be attributed to surgical trauma.

Posterior injuries may include:

Posterior capsule
Posterior cruciate ligament
Medial collateral ligament
Medial meniscus
Fibular collateral ligament
Peroneal nerve
Anterior cruciate ligament

Here again, my contention is that the knee is supported by a group of ligaments making a solid cuff, or pocket, to surround and stabilize the knee.

Injuries to the cruciate ligament are:

Anterior cruciate, most commonly in medial side injuries
Posterior cruciate, most commonly in lateral side injuries

Usually they occur in combination with some other injury to the knee. I don't subscribe wholly to Dr. KENNEDY'S statement that a truly isolated injury of the anterior cruciate ligament must be very rare. I have found these isolated injuries in the course of doing an arthrotomy on the knee for something other than the cruciate, if it is an unrecognized cruciate injury. So you must at least have the meniscus injury or you would not have been operating the patient. But the meniscus injury will probably have some damage to the medial ligament and medial capsular fibers. The question as to whether it is an isolated injury is rather futile; I don't think it makes all that much difference whether we call it isolated or not. I prefer to call it unrecognized, which I think is a little more realistic.

Method of Examination

As for the actual examination, the following factors should be considered:

History
Time, place and manner
Inspection
Palpation
Manipulation
X-ray

I think the history is very important. In many instances you can make a diagnosis from the history alone. Although an examination is necessary, if you trust your patient's integrity and he gives you a pretty straightforward story, you can probably tell pretty well about his instability. One of my patients was actually able to supply me with a photograph taken at the time he was injured. Of course, I did not have the picture at the time I first examined him. This Oklahoma player was hurt during one of the Orange Bowl games when he tried to catch the ball. This was an acute injury which, theoretically, we are not discussing here. We are talking more about the results of these injuries. The player was able to tell me exactly what happened. He said his foot was fixed as he twisted around to catch the ball, the knee was a little

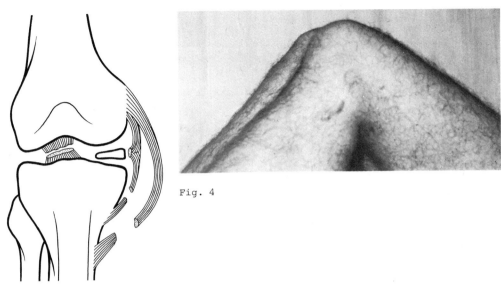

Fig. 3

Fig. 4

Fig. 3. Classic injury: Note superficial layer and deep layer of medial collateral ligament torn near tibial attachment with ruptured medial meniscus and completely torn anterior cruciate ligament [2]

Fig. 4. Posterior sag. profile of the left (nearer) knee sags backward compared to the normal right knee [1]

bit flexed and he was turning away from the fixed foot. He was just then hit at the side of the knee. He fell to the ground, his leg a little off to one side; the official came over and pulled his leg straight. He was unable to walk on it. From that narration you can be sure there is medial collateral damage, involving possibly also the anterior cruciate (Fig. 3). So, the history is important. What this boy actually had was a torn anterior cruciate ligament, with the short capsular fibers and the long medial collateral fibers off the tibia; there was also meniscus rupture. You can see, it pays to talk to the patient.

The time of the examination is quite important. It should be done as soon as you can get the patient to where you can do an adequate examination. This is just as true in reconstruction as it is in acute injuries.

I can tell you the manner of my examination, but that does not necessarily mean that this must be your method. You should, however, follow a regular pattern of examination since you otherwise very likely may forget to include some parts. You need to get the patient's clothes off; you can't examine an unstable knee if you haven't taken the patient's pants off. I have had the patient ask why since he never had this done before when he was examined. It is important to have him stand up to observe both legs and to compare one leg with the other, not impeded by a lot of taping, clothes, or anything else.

An overall inspection should be made. Observe the patient walking. See what he looks like with or without crutches. Stand him against the wall and take a look at him. Is there an obvious deformity? Is there obvious swelling? Does he have scars on his skin? Have him stand perpendicular to the wall with his weight on both legs and then have him raise one leg, then the other. With the leg hanging off the table, examine the position of the patella and the general condition of the leg. With the patient supine, notice the contour of both legs with the knees at 90°. Does the tibia hang backward, suggesting posterior cruciate and posterior capsular redundancy (Fig. 4)? you can tell this just by observing the patient rather than touching him.

Following observation, palpation is an important part of the examination to determine whether there is effusion or hemarthrosis, swelling, or increased temperature. Check particularly for location of tenderness, if any. Tenderness is more consistently at the site of involvement than any other place. Have the patient kick his leg up and down to see if there is crepitation under the patella or in the retinaculum. Try to locate where the crepitation actually is. Is it increased or decreased by loading? Have the patient squat to see if this is painful. Determine where it hurts. Is the knee unstable? Can he come up on the one leg or the other? All these things add to the sum total of your information about the patient.

Not until we have concluded the inspection and palpation do we usually manipulate the leg for instability. Having checked the active range of motion, note any restriction of flexion or extension. Ask the patient if he can voluntarily move his knee into an abnormal position, such as rotating his tibia forward or backward. Then make these same tests yourself. With the knee in extension, i.e., the position in which the posterior capsule is tight, note whether there is any medial or lateral rotatory or any anteroposterior abnormal motion. With the leg in complete extension, place lateral stress on the leg (Fig. 5a). If the knee opens up on the inner side demonstrating medial side instability, then the medial capsular ligaments, the medial posterior capsule,

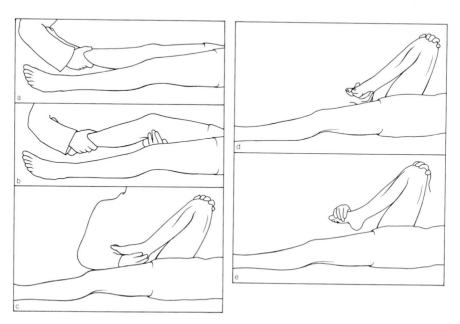

Fig. 5a-e. a Lateral motion checked with the knee extended. b Lateral motion checked with the knee flexed. c Forced flexion to determine whether there is pain or snapping with the leg neutral. d Forced flexion with the leg internally rotated. e Forced flexion with the leg externally rotated

and probably the anterior and posterior cruciate ligaments are torn. If you flex the knee a little bit and make the same tests, you now eliminate the posterior capsule; this will open up quite materially without any damage to the posterior capsule or the posterior cruciate (Fig. 5b). It is a much more favorable condition to have increased instability in a little flexion than it is to have instability with the knee extended because with the knee extended you are bound to have pretty serious intrinsic injuries in the knee.

With the patient supine, check the knee in complete flexion with the foot straight (Fig. 5c); then in complete flexion with the foot internally rotated (Fig. 5d); than with the foot externally rotated. With the foot internally rotated and adducted, note any unusual movement or sound when moving from the extreme flexed position out to complete extension. This should also be repeated when the leg is externally rotated (Fig. 5e).

It is very important to check rotation of the tibia on the femur and particularly the axis of rotation. Should the axis of rotation be in the center of the tibia, if the medial side comes forward, the lateral side will go back, and vice versa. If the axis of rotation moves to either side, the opposite side will rotate, but the side of the tibia to which the actual rotation has migrated will not advance. In taking a stress X-ray with the knee in extension and a second stress X-ray with the knee in flexion, you can readily see with the posterior capsule intact (extension position) that there is not much opening up; however, with the knee in flexion, it may open up quite markedly (Fig. 6). You cannot have anteromedial rotatory instability when you are not

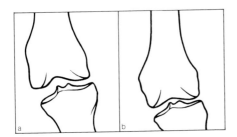

Fig. 6. Drawings from X-rays of stressed (a) knee in flexed position and (b) knee extended. Note the markedly greater amount of opening up when the posterior capsule is eliminated in a

having posterolateral rotatory instability unless the axis of the center of rotation has changed. The center of rotation has moved over toward the side which does not shift forward or backward, but remains neutral. The opposite side will come forward or backward. The most common form of rotatory instability I see is anteromedial rotatory instability. To do this, the center of rotation has to leave the posterior cruciate ligament and move to the lateral side. That does not necessarily mean that the posterior cruciate ligament is torn. Rotatory instability can be quite complex, and often the exact pathology may differ from case to case.

To test for anteroposterior instability, I like to test for the drawer sign by having the patient sit on the edge of the table with his legs dangling freely at 90° (Fig. 7). Check the good side first, then the pathologic side. Sit on a stool in front of the patient, locking his foot between your knees with his foot straight ahead. Grasp the calf of his leg and pull forward, then push backward, to see whether there is forward and backward motion. Then put the foot in external rotation and check the same motion. Then put the foot in internal rotation and check the same motion for the amount of instability. I don't like to

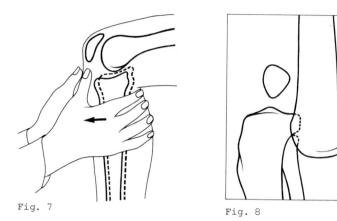

Fig. 7

Fig. 8

Fig. 7. The drawer maneuver used to check anteroposterior motion [1]

Fig. 8. Drawing of "as is" X-ray of completely dislocated knee. This patient sustained a severe sprain (third degree), and it is obvious that there must be extensive ligamentous damage

make this test with the patient supine because he almost automatically tightens up the hamstrings to keep the foot from slipping. Tight hamstrings will completely eliminate a positive sign and invalidate the test.

X-ray is extremely important. X-ray technicians are trained to take certain positions routinely. I prefer to see what the leg looks like without anyone touching it, so we just lay the leg down on the X-ray plate without support and take an "as is" X-ray of it. Sometimes this will be very enlightening and may show gross deformity involving a good deal of ligament damage (Fig. 8). An X-ray made with the leg in complete extension and not supported may indicate almost as much damage as the X-ray of a leg with a complete dislocation (Fig. 9). Unsupported,

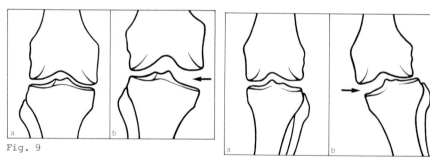

Fig. 9

Fig. 10

Fig. 9a and b. Complete dislocation. a Positioned anteroposterior view showing an apparently normal knee. b Drawing of X-ray of same knee when unsupported. Notice the wide gap on the medial side

Fig. 10a and b. Injury to medial collateral ligament. a Neutral anteroposterior view. b Position of abduction of leg on thigh. Arrow indicates increased tibiofemoral joint space. The lateral side collapses from the normal space at a to about one-half the space at b. The total amount of instability would be the sum of the difference between the two sides

the knee may sag open with the leg in complete extension; this means that both cruciates, the medial posterior capsule, and all the medial components must be gone. When that same leg is positioned as for a normal anteroposterior view with someone holding it, it may be quite negative. You can show that pathology with stress X-ray, but I think that if you can get this sort of film without stress, you get much more information about what has happened. Therefore, we take "as is" antero-posterior, lateral, oblique, and silhouette X-ray before we do any stress X-rays.

Interpretation of a stress X-ray needs some explanation too (Fig. 10). The combination of medial and lateral instability is much more serious than either one or the other alone. A lot of apparent lateral instability demonstrated may be from collapse of the opposite side, as well as opening up of the side being tested. We measure in millimeters but we do not have any fixed tables. We actually compare the change from compressed to stretched, i.e., the medial side compressed 4 mm and stretched to 8 mm equals 4 mm instability.

I do not routinely take an arthrogram or an arthroscopic examination because they ordinarily will be negative. Neither of these tests are informative about chronic instability and certainly are not necessary for diagnosis. We do use X-rays on the North American continent, but sometimes we do not use them very judiciously. X-rays may show fractures or displacements. The site of ligament injury may be indicated by a flake of bone or exogenous ossification. This may quite simplify the operation; it may indicate the location of the lesion so that you are able to freshen up the bone and just tuck the fragment back down. This may be much simpler than many of the reconstructions that we have to do. I have been quoted as saying that the X-ray is not important in ligament injuries, but that is not true. It is extremely important. You do not, however, need an X-ray to diagnose instability.

I recently saw a 9 year old girl who had had a bicycle injury 6 months before and who now had a painful and restricted knee. The original X-ray was negative; the doctor had prescribed neither support nor any treatment besides rest. Examination showed there as anteroposterior instability with a positive anterior drawer sign. We re-X-rayed her knee and found that the top of the tibia had been pulled loose and was angulated upward 45° which checked her flexion and relaxed the anterior cruciate ligament (Fig. 11).

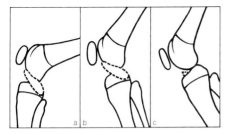

Fig. 11. Drawing of X-ray of avulsed upper tibia. (a) Acute injury with a large frag-ment of upper tibia avulsed by the anterior cruciate. (b) Four months later, fragment in the same position, and the knee at maximum extension. Range of motion, 30°. (c) Two months after removal of the fragment, some recurrance of ossification. Range (9 months post-injury and 5 months postoperative) is 20° to 90°. This disability could have been prevented by adequate early treatment

Surgery revealed that the bone was pulled up by the anterior cruciate ligament. Reconstruction was easy and successful. On the basis of this example, one can see that repeat X-rays are a must if symptoms persist. Again, it is important also to compare the damaged leg with the normal.

We get back to where we started, remembering that diagnosis is the most important factor in knee instability. Almost anyone can be taught to do a certain method of reconstruction, but the most important thing is to diagnose at the start what is wrong with the knee and then try to decide whether or not reconstruction is necessary. Proper treatment depends upon proper diagnosis.

References

1. O'DONOGHUE, D.H.: Treatment of injuries to athletes. 3rd. Ed. Philadelphia: Saunders, 1976
2. O'DONOGHUE, D.H.: Surgical treatment of fresh injuries to the major ligaments of the knee. J. Bone Joint Surg. 32A, 4, 725 (1950)

6. Assessment of Chronic Ligamentous Instability Using Arthrography, Arthroscopy, and Anesthesia

M. E. Blazina

A definite inter-relationship exists between four major groups of pathology encountered in knee surgery, i.e., lesions of the menisci, ligamentous instability, patellar tracking problems, and articular cartilage damage (Fig. 1). To segregate one's thinking solely to one of these major components without thinking of the others ignores the totality approach to knee derangements.

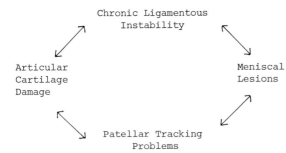

Fig. 1. Inter-relationship between meniscal pathology and chronic ligamentous instability

There are some surgeons who are concerned only with removal of menisci. It has certainly been emphasized that a distinct inter-relationship exists between meniscal pathology and chronic ligamentous instability. If one removes a meniscus and the patient has significant residual ligamentous instability, the functional result will be unsatisfactory, and there is a distinct possibility that further surgery will be necessary. Likewise, if one concentrates on other areas but ignores the patella, then the results also may be unsatisfactory. There has been a tendency on the part of knee replacement surgeons to discount the importance of the patellofemoral joint. Also, parenthetically, we all recognize the importance of adequate extensor mechanism rehabilitation following knee surgery.

Insofar as articular cartilage damage is concerned, we try by our stabilizing procedures to prevent or slow down degenerative processes. On the other hand, there must be a point at which the articular cartilage damage is of such a sufficient degree that stabilizing procedures alone will be fruitless and we must consider replacement or arthrodesis.

Diagnosis Using Normal Clinical Methods

In assessing a knee with chronic ligamentous instability, we have
developed a <u>check-out</u> list which attempts to determine as definitively
as possible not only all the components of instability, but also the
status of the menisci, the extensor mechanism, patellofemoral articu-
lations, and the articular cartilage of the medial and lateral compartments (Table 1). Everyone would agree that the basic approach
always has been and always will be a detailed history and a thorough

Table 1. Check-List for Assessment of Chronic Ligamentous Instability

I. *Menisci*

Normal?	Abnormal?	
Torn? Where?	Not torn?	
In?	Out?	
Completely out?		Partially out?
Regenerated?		Degree of regeneration?

II. *Articular Cartilages*

Medial compartment - lateral compartment
Medial femoral condyle - medial tibial condyle
Lateral femoral condyle - lateral tibial condyle

III. *Extensor Mechanism*

Alignment
Stability
Articular cartilages
  Patellofemoral groove
Plicae

IV. *Ligaments*

Anteromedial-, anterior-posterior-neutral, and anterolateral
Posteromedial, posteroanterior-neutral, and posterolateral
Valgus - varus
Recurvatum

physical examination. Routine X-rays should not only include the standard anteroposterior and lateral views, but also the intercondylar
notch and patellar tangential views. On occasion, oblique views may
be helpful. During the past decade a certain element of controversy
has arisen over the relative efficacies of arthrography and arthroscopy and their relevancy to the study of the deranged knee. First
of all, we should like to point out that sophistication becomes inherent in the study of knee problems. At an elementary level, just as
in beginning golf, one can get by with a minimum number of tools or
clubs. On the other hand, at an advanced level, one needs and uses
<u>all</u> the tools or clubs allowed or available. Secondly, as has been
demonstrated so often in other areas of study in the past, specialized
techniques such as arthrography and arthroscopy art not substitutes
for the basic approaches, but are used either for further information
or for confirmatory techniques for initial impressions. Thirdly,
arthrography and arthroscopy are not necessarily doing the same thing
in different ways. Arthrography may provide information unavailable
or difficult to obtain with the arthroscope but may also have definite
limitations. Likewise, arthroscopy may provide information unavailable

or difficult to obtain with arthrography but may have limitations as well. An attempt to delineate the capabilities of each technique will be pointed out further on in the discussion.

Insofar as the status of the menisci is concerned, we would like to know the information given in Table 1. If the menisci are torn, would partial meniscectomy alone be helpful? Some of this information may be obtained from a review of previous operative reports or at the time of physical examination, but in neither case necessarily so.

Insofar as the status of the articular cartilages is concerned, we would like to know whether any damage is present and if so, the degree and extent of that articular cartilage damage. A little bit of roughening and a completely denuded condyle represent definitely different degrees of damage and may influence our attitudes towards the efficacy of our planned ligamentous reconstruction. Dr. O'DONOGHUE showed a case with posterolateral instability. The X-rays of that case showed narrowing of the medial compartment. It would be very important to know the exact degree of involvement of that compartment, since the ultimate prognosis may ride on that.

Insofar as the extensor mechanism is concerned, in the past it has not received enough attention. One can have underlying patellar instability complicated by ligamentous injury, or one can have an acquired patellar instability secondary to ligamentous injury. We are extremely interested in the status of the articular cartilages of the patellofemoral articulation and have pointed out in another discussion under what a mechanical disadvantage the patella is working in cases of posterior instability with a tibial drop-back. We are also interested in the cartilage if a synovial plica exists.

Insofar as the ligamentous instability itself is concerned, it is important that we delineate and correct all the major components of instability. Dr. KENNEDY has already pointed out that if three major components are present and only two components are corrected, the result will be unsatisfactory.

In evaluating meniscal lesions, articular cartilage damage, the extensor mechanism, and the major components of ligamentous instability, it would be our feeling that we could use the added help derived from arthrography, arthroscopy, and examination under anesthesia.

Diagnostic Use of Arthrography

Arthrography, as you know, is an old technique which was almost abandoned after World War II, probably because the dyes injected into the knee at that time were very irritating. In 1960 in Los Angeles only one radiologist was performing arthrography, and he was doing pneumoarthrography. After spending some time in Sweden, certain radiologists in Los Angeles began to use the newer radio-opaque dyes with increasing success and minimal morbidity. At the present time we perhaps are becoming too dependent on arthrography. We except it to make a diagnosis for us and have been reluctant to recognize its limitations (Table 2).

Insofar as the menisci are concerned, arthrography is very helpful in its own right in evaluating the posterior horn of the medial meniscus in an unoperated knee. Correlated with the clinical impressions, it

Table 2. Arthrogram

I.   For injuries to menisci

  A. Useful in diagnosing

    Lesions of medial meniscus (unoperated knee),
    especially posterior horn

    Some lesions of lateral meniscus

  B. Of no use in diagnosing

    Midportion lesions of lateral meniscus

    Early cleavage lesions of menisci

II. For injuries to articular cartilages of no diagnostic use

III. For injuries to extensor mechanism of no diagnostic use

IV. For injuries to ligaments

  A. Of some use in diagnosing
     Peripheral capsular lesions
     Collateral ligament avulsions

  B. Of very little use in diagnosing
     Status of cruciate ligaments

---

may be helpful in avoiding removing a normal meniscus or on the other
hand may keep us from leaving in a medial meniscus with a posterior
horn tear.

Arthrography may be helpful in evaluating the lateral meniscus, but
not to the degree suggested by arthrography enthusiasts. It has been
our impression that arthrography is helpful in evaluating the lateral
meniscus about 50% of the time. It may fail to reveal a lateral meniscus which subsequently is proven to be definitely torn, or it may
lead one to suspect a lateral meniscus tear when it does not exist.

Arthrography is not helpful in evaluating early cleavage lesions of
the meniscus and may lead to great confusion and the profoundest
misimpressions when utilized in evaluating a post-meniscectomy situation. The arthrographic impression that a very large fragment has
been left in posteriorly may be completely unsubstantiated at subsequent surgery. We forget that the dye may not be able to enter a
scarred area! An arthrographic diagnosis of a retained fragment has
serious medical malpractice implications in our state of California.
In the same vein, it is very difficult to evaluate meniscal regeneration. Some arthrograms may appear to show extensive meniscal regeneration which is not substantiated at arthroscopy or arthrotomy.

Arthrography helps very little in evaluating the extensor mechanism.
Occasionally, the dye may outline a radiolucent chondral fracture or
chondral loose body. One may also attempt to evaluate the apparent
thickness of the articular cartilages of the patellofemoral articulation.

Arthrography may be of some help in evaluating ligamentous injuries.
Dr. O'DONOGHUE has shown a slide depicting extravasation of dye up
along the medial capsule to the medial femoral epicondyle. This finding is suggestive of a deep medial capsular ligament tear in its

meniscofemoral portion and helps localize the site of the actual
lesion. A great deal of effort has been spent in arthrographic evaluation of cruciate ligament lesions, including lateral laminagrams
and stress films. Perhaps one can differentiate an intact cruciate
from an absent cruciate, but as noted in other discussions, it is
important definitively to differentiate such problems as a nonfunctioning attenuated intact cruciate and a partial tear. Perhaps this
necessity is too much to expect from arthrography.

As described above, arthrography may be of some help in determining
the thickness of the articular cartilages in the medial and lateral
compartments. But it cannot help us in determining the type of articular lesion actually existing and really cannot evaluate its extent.

Diagnostic Use of Arthroscopy

Arthroscopy has proven to be a very useful tool in assessing knee
derangements. It is not a substitute for arthrography and should also
not be over-utilized (Table 3).

Table 3. Arthroscopy

I.   For injuries to menisci

    A. Useful in diagnosing

       Displaced cartilage tears

       Lesions of anterior 2/3 of medial meniscus of
       lateral meniscus

    B. Of limited use in diagnosing

       Posterior horn tears of medial meniscus

II. For injuries to articular cartilages

    A. Of great use in diagnosing

       Lesions of medial femoral condyle, medial tibial condyle,
       lateral femoral condyle, lateral tibial condyle

III. For injuries to extensor mechanism

    A. Of great use in diagnosing

       Lesions of patellar and femoral groove
       Synovial plicae

IV. For injuries to ligaments

    A. Of great use in diagnosing

       Anterior cruciate ligament lesions

    B. Of limited use in diagnosing

       Peripheral capsular lesions

       Posterior cruciate ligament lesions

With the arthroscope we can easily visualize the anterior two-thirds of the medial meniscus and the entire lateral meniscus. It has its limitations in evaluating the posterior horn of the medial meniscus (clinical evaluation and arthrography will help us there); also an early cleavage lesion may not be seen. Flap tears are readily noted and regenerated menisci or residual tags can be seen. With the recent emphasis on performing a partial meniscectomy, the arthroscope has come to the fore as an aid in this determination. Also, it aids in determing the feasibility of concentrating all of our work on just one side.

Arthroscopy allows us to evaluate the status of the cruciate ligaments, especially the anterior cruciate ligament. We can foresee the time when it may help provide useful information in evaluating the actual functional capabilities of the anterior cruciate ligament, especially the attentuated or partially torn ligaments.

Arthroscopy is of great help in evaluating the status of the articular cartilages of the medial and lateral compartments and of the status of the articular cartilages of the patellofemoral articulation. The degree of damage can be assessed fairly accurately. Free-floating chondral loose bodies and synovial plica may be visualized and removed.

Examination Under Anesthesia

Lastly, we should like to emphasize the importantce of examination of the knee under anesthesia (Table 4). Certainly, if arthroscopy is being done with the patient asleep, a golden opportunity exists to evaluate range of motion and compartmental clicks and to assess accurately ligamentous instability. All too often, an arthroscopic report makes no

Table 4. Anesthesia

I.   For injuries to menisci

    A. Of some use in diagnosing

       Compartment clicks

II. For injuries to articular cartilages

    A. Of some use in diagnosing

       Compartment crepitus

III. For injuries to extensor mechanism

    A. Of some use in diagnosing

       Tight vastus lateralis

       Patellar hypermobility

IV. For injuries to ligaments

    A. Of great use in diagnosing

       Anterolateral instability

       Posteroanterior-neutral instability

       Posterolateral instability

    B. Of some use in diagnosing

       Anteromedial instability

       Anteroposterior-neutral instability

       Valgus - varus instability

       Recurvatum

---

mention of the above phenomena. Also, at the time of actual surgery, one should pre-operatively evaluate the knee and after removing a torn meniscus, another ligamentous evaluation should be performed. Dr. SLOCUM has pointed out that a jammed knee may portray a false sense of stability and after removal of the jamming factor the knee may be quite unstable. Finally, one should judiciously test the knee after ligamentous reconstruction to ascertain the degree of improvement obtained.

In summary, the added techniques of arthrography, arthroscopy, and examination under anesthesia are not substitutes for a careful initial examination. Also they are complementary to each other - not competitive.

Discussion

SCHULITZ: Professor HIPP, what's your opinion on arthrography and arthroscopy?

HIPP: So far we have not performed arthroscopy, but only arthrography. If carried out accurately, arthrography can give decisive clues. However, we feel that arthrography is not carried out selectively enough. My collegue Dr. KARPF treated 100 patients who had been accurately arthrographed by the same examiner in a series of examinations. Dr. KARPF will relate his experience.

KARPF: We were able to diagnose 95 of these cases by clinical examination, whereas arthrography was only positive in 84 cases. We believe that arthrography is not necessary for the purely meniscal injury. Among the 100 cases mentioned above we had 42 combined cases, i.e. anteromedial and anterolateral rotatory instabilities. Since surgery has to be done in these cases anyhow, arthrography is only necessary in a selected number of them, for example, after meniscectomy.

BÖHLER: I would like to emphasize the value of arthroscopy. We feel that it is much more important than Professor HIPP thought. I would like to quote the results of ERIKSSON. For acute damages of the knee joint, on the basis of clinical examination he made the correct diagnosis of the complete complex of the lesions in 35% of the patients. With examination under anaesthesia it was around 60%, and with arthroscopy nearly 90%. We have had the same experience, especially in relation to cartilaginous lesions.

7. Procedures Utilized for Chronic Ligamentous Instability of the Knee, Including a Statistical Review

M. E. Blazina

Statistical Review

A review of knee surgery in general reveals that about 25% of the procedures are utilized as attempts to correct chronic ligamentous instability (Table 1).

Table 1. Ligamentous reconstruction procedures

1. Posteromedial capsular reefing	1074
2. Pes anserinus transfer	713
3. Anteromedial capsular reefing	291
4. Vastus medialis transposition	282
5. Proximal medial collateral ligament advancement	151
6. Modified Ellison procedure	108
7. Ellison procedure	92
8. Medial collateral ligament reconstruction (O'DONOGHUE)	75
9. Posterolateral capsular reefing	66
10. McIntosh-Galway procedure (anterolateral instability)	63
11. Prosthetic anterior cruciate ligament	57
12. Anterolateral capsular reefing	48
13. Biceps transfer to lateral femoral epicondyle	35
14. Anterior cruciate ligament reconstruction	33
15. Lateral cruciate ligament reconstruction	29
16. Prosthetic medial collateral ligament	22
17. Posterior cruciate ligament reconstruction	21
18. Prosthetic posterior cruciate ligament	18
19. Secondary pes anserinus transfer	18
20. Reverse modified Ellison procedure	16
21. Semimembranosus transfer to medial femoral epicondyle	13
22. Medial collateral ligament	11
23. Biceps forward	8
24. McIntosh posterolateral reconstruction	7
25. Secondary medialis transposition	7
26. Anterior transposition of semitendinosus	6
	3264 (24%)

Table 2. Relationship of procedures to operations

No. of operations = 5,578
No. of procedures = 13,699
Procedures/operation = 2.5

We feel that it is important to differentiate between "operations" and "procedures" (Table 2). In a single operation more than one procedure may be performed, and any one of these procedures may have significant bearing on the ultimate prognosis. As an example, to talk about a large group of "medial meniscectomies" without discussing the concomitant procedures that were utilized, really negates the true impact of such a study. "Medial meniscectomy" alone is a much different operation than "medial meniscectomy plus anterior cruciate ligament reconstruction." We have had a great deal of difficulty trying to interpret the meaning of Professor SMILLIE'S extremely large series of over 8000 mensicectomies.

Incidentally, medial meniscectomy and lateral meniscectomy stand by far in the forefront insofar as the frequency of types of procedures is concerned (Table 3). As a reflection, if someone would really like to revolutionize knee surgery, the greatest impact would be delivered by developing the capability of inserting a new meniscus at the time of meniscectomy.

Table 3. Procedures

1. Medial meniscectomy	2343
2. Lateral meniscectomy	1113
3. Posteromedial capsular reefing	1074
4. Vastus medialis transposition	848
5. Pes anserinus transfer	713
6. Vastus lateralis release	706
7. Patellaplasty	595
8. Removal of loose bodies	467
9. Chondroplasty of medial femoral condyle	383
10. Transfer of tibial tubercule	305
11. Anteromedial capsular reefing	291
12. Secondary medial meniscectomy	277
13. Excision of tag of anterior cruicate ligament	223
14. Medial patellar retinaculum advancement	221
15. Medial collateral ligament	218
16. Roux-Goldthwaite	197
17. Chondroplasty of lateral femoral condyle	189
18. Partial synovnovectomy	189
19. Proximal medial collateral ligament advancement	151
20. Medial compartment replacement	142

Besides primary lesions of the menisci, another procedure is described in Table 3 which is called "secondary medial meniscectomy," performed 277 times. All secondary medial meniscectomies do not connote a removal of a retained fragment; the greater number of them relate to the removal of a regenerated medial meniscus at the time of a subsequent operation, be it for whatever coexisting problems.

At present, we do not know the incidence of reoperation following medial meniscectomy. Some of the procedures are related to ligamentous instability, such as the pes anserinus transfer. One can also note "excision of a tag of the anterior cruciate ligament" performed 223 times! One wonders about the natural history of these cases.

Some of the procedures are related to patellar tracking problems, such as vastus lateralis release. Other procedures relate to articular cartilage damage, such as chondroplasty of the medial femoral condyle.

Table 1 represents a specific description of ligamentous reconstruction procedures performed. Here one notes besides pes anserinus transfer, such procedures as proximal medial collateral ligament advancement, the Ellison procedure, biceps tendon transfer to the lateral femoral epicondyle, etc. We would hope that this list will serve as a prelude for following discussion.

Description of Some Procedures

Accompanying this list are some figures depicting certain procedures, especially the Ellison procedure.

60

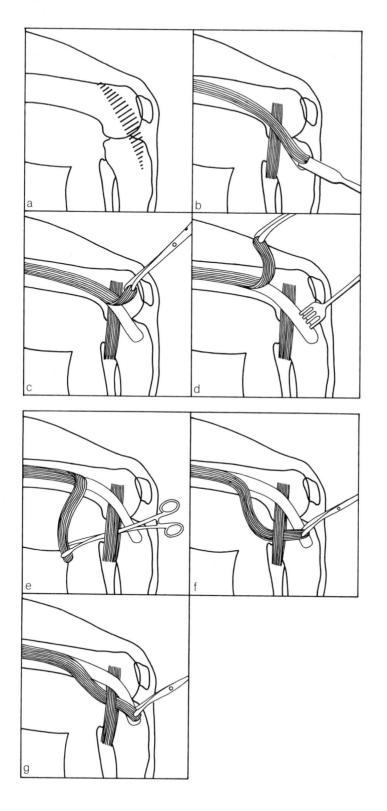

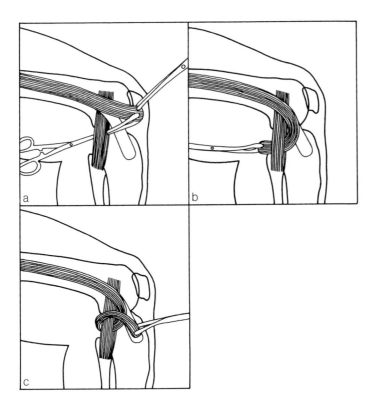

Fig. 2a-c. Modified Ellison procedure. a The curved Kocher is passed from backwards to forwards under the lateral collateral ligament to grasp the button of bone and the attached strip of iliotibial band. b The button of bone with the attached strip of iliotibial band is passed under the lateral collateral ligament from anterior to posterior exiting superiorly near the lateral femoral epicondyle. c With the lower leg in external rotation and the knee in flexion, the button of bone is refixated to the original site of origin at Gerdy's tubercle (here with barbed staples). The stay sutures are brought forward and sutured to the anterior edge of the lateral collateral ligament. The defect in the iliotibial band is closed

◁ ───

Fig. 1a-d. Ellison procedure. a Incision along anterolateral aspect of knee from above lateral femoral epicondyle distally across joint line to just beyond Gerdy's tubercle. b A strip of iliotibial band approximately 1.5-2.0 cm wide is detached distally along with a button of bone from Gerdy's tubercle. c The strip of iliotibial band is dissected free from the underlying tissues proximally up to the level of the intermuscular septum. d Vertical incisions are made in the lateral capsule anterior and posterior to the lateral collateral ligament. The lateral collateral ligament is freed from the underlying popliteus tendon. Stay sutures may be placed in the posterolateral capsules to be brought forward later

Fig. 1e-g. e A curved Kocher is passed under the lateral collateral ligament from forwards to backwards (i.e., in the space between the lateral collateral ligament and the popliteus tendon) and used to grasp the button of bone attached to the strip of iliotibial band. f The strip of iliotibial band is then passed under the lateral collateral ligament from posterior to anterior. g With the lower leg in external rotation and the knee in flexion, the button of bone is fixated (here with barbed staples) to the upper lateral tibia anterior and distal to Gerdy's tubercle. The stay sutures in the posterolateral capsule are then brought forward and sutured to the anterior aspect of the lateral collateral ligament

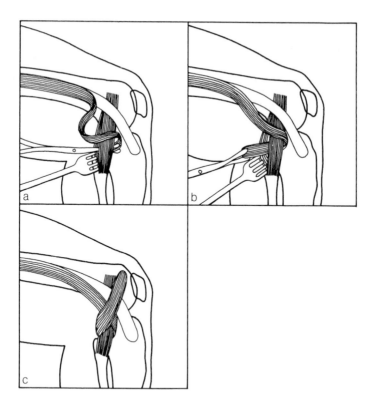

Fig. 3. a The curved Kocher is passed from backwards to forwards under the lateral collateral ligament to grasp the button of bone and the attached strip of iliotibial band. b The button of bone with the attached strip of iliotibial band is passed under the lateral collateral ligament from anterior to posterior, exiting inferiorly near the fibular attachment of the lateral collateral ligament. c With the lower leg in internal rotation and the knee flexed, the button of bone is fixated to the lateral femoral epicondyle as far anteriorly as possible without encroaching on the articular surface or the femoral origin of the popliteus tendon. A small trough may be made in the area of designated fixation to prevent the development of a protuberance. The stay sutures in the posterolateral capsule are brought forward and sutured to the anterior edge of the lateral collateral ligament. The defect in the iliotibial band is closed

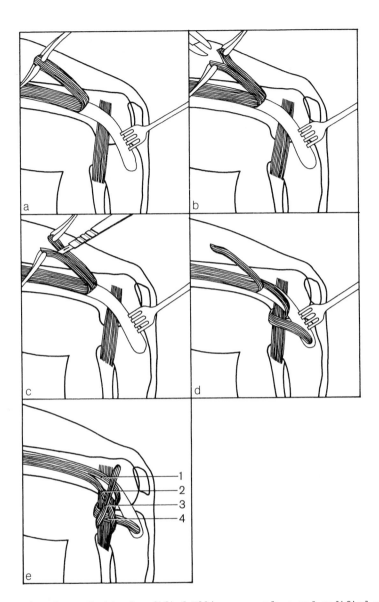

Fig. 4a-e. Combined modified Ellison procedure and modified reverse Ellison procedure. a The button of bone (with the strip of iliotibial band attached) is grasped on each side with a Lahey clamp. b The button of bone is cut in two longitudinally with a bone cutter. c With a scalpel, two longitudinal strips of iliotibial band are developed along with buttons of bone at the distal ends. d With the curved Kocher, the most anterior strip is passed under the lateral collateral ligament from forwards to backwards exiting at the lateral femoral epicondyle. This strip eventually will run back down to the area of Gerdy's tubercle. e The second strip (i.e., the most posterior strip) is also passed under the lateral collateral ligament from forwards to backwards, exiting near the fibular attachment of the lateral collateral ligament. 1. This strip eventually will run up to anterior aspect of the lateral femoral epicondyle. 2. With the lower leg in external rotation and the knee in flexion, strip No. 1 (i.e., the anterior strip) is fixated back down to Gerdy's tubercle. 3. Then, with the lower leg in internal rotation and the knee in flexion, strip No. 2 (i.e., the posterior strip) is fixated to the anterior aspect of the lateral femoral epicondyle. 4. The stay sutures are sutured to the anterior aspect of the lateral collateral ligament. 5. The defect in the iliotibial band is closed

Semimembranosus Transfer to Medial Femoral Epicondyle

1. Oblique incision extending from medial femoral epicondyle distally across joint line to region of pes anserinus.

2. Posteromedial capsule incised just posterior to medial collateral ligament, extended inferiorly to expose semimembranosus tendon.

3. Semimembranosus tendon insertion into upper tibia anteriorly is detached underneath the medial collateral ligament.

4. Semimembranosus tendon is freed up proximally without detaching attachments to posterior oblique ligament or posteromedial capsule.

5. Stay sutures placed in posteromedial capsule.

6. With lower leg in external rotation and knee in flexion, semimembranosus tendon is fixated to medial femoral epicondyle as far anteriorly as possible.

7. Posteromedial capsule is reefed utilizing the stay sutures.

Posterior Cruciate Ligament Reconstruction Utilizing Medial Meniscus

1. Oblique incision extending from medial femoral epicondyle distally across joint line to region of pes anserinus.

2. Anteromedial capsular incision. Anterior horn of medial meniscus detached and medial meniscus detached to just beyond posterior limb of medial collateral ligament.

3. Posteromedial capsular incision just posterior to medial collateral ligament.

a. Medial meniscus brought out through this aperture and posterior capsular attachments detached, leaving medial meniscus attached to posterior horn in intercondylar region.

b. A test to see that medial meniscus will displace easily and fully into intercondylar notch.

c. Stay sutures in posteromedial capsule.

4. Drill hole made in medial femoral condyle, exiting in intercondylar notch at site of origin of posterior cruciate ligament from femur.

5. Medial meniscus pulled into the above hole and fixated with sutures placed through periosteum at medial femoral epicondyle. Fixation is performed with tibia being brought forward and knee flexed.

6. Stay sutures in posteromedial capsule utilized to reef the posteromedial capsule.

Posterior Cruciate Ligament Reconstruction Utilizing the Medial Head of the Gastrocnemius

1. Oblique incision extending from medial femoral epicondyle distally across joint line to region of pes anserinus.

2. Anteromedial capsular incision.

3. Posteromedial capsular incision just posterior to medial collateral ligament.

4. Medial strip of medial head of gastrocnemius tendon detached from femur as high up as possible.

5. Aperture made in posteromedial capsule near midline. Run medial head of gastrocnemius through this aperture, exiting inside joint near site of tibial origin of posterior cruciate ligament.

6. Drill hole made in medial femoral condyle, exiting in intercondylar notch at site of origin of posterior cruciate ligament from femur.

7. Strip of medial head of gastrocnemius pulled into above hole and fixated with sutures placed through periosteum at medial femoral epicondyle. Fixation is performed with tibia brought forward and knee flexed.

8. Posteromedial capsule reefed.

Biceps Tendon Transfer to Lateral Femoral Epicondyle

1. Incision along anterolateral aspect of knee from above lateral femoral epicondyle distally across joint line to just beyond Gerdy's tubercle, curving there slightly posteriorly.

2. Biceps tendon identified and freed up as far proximally as possible.

3. Anterior 4/5 of biceps tendon detached proximally and strip of tendon developed distally all the way to the fibular styloid process, leaving the strip firmly attached to the fibular styloid process.

4. Two 1/4 in. drill holes are made in the lateral femoral epicondyle vertically, leaving a substantial plate of bone between the two holes. These holes are made as far anteriorly as possible avoiding the femoral origin of the popliteus tendon.

5. The biceps tendon is passed through the inferior drill hole, then through the superior drill hole, and then turned back down and sutured to itself under tension with the knee in varus and the lower leg in internal rotation.

8. Reconstruction for Medial Instability of the Knee.
Surgical Technique

D. H. O'Donoghue

Advisability of Knee Reconstruction

In dealing with acute knee ligament injuries, the main thing is to
find the torn ligaments and to put them together again. Knee reconstruction, on the contrary, is a salvage operation. The questions to
be answered are: Who should have a ligament reconstruction? Why should
it be done? When should it be done? Where should it be done? Who should
do it?

Who should have a ligament reconstruction? There is a difference of opinion
here; I think that is a healthy sign because each case must be strictly
individualized, and the patient must be very much aware of his share
of the problem. If he is the least bit hesitant about the operation,
then it is better not to do it, because this is a sort of "last chance"
thing. The surgeon doesn't just look at the knee and say, "We will
operate you tomorrow." At least, I do not think he should.

The patient should be constitutionally fit for it. The first thing you
should determine is the difference between instability and disability,
as Dr. BLAZINA explained in the preceeding article. A patient may have
a considerable amount of instability and not actually have much disability. You should not put this patient through a long program of
surgery and rehabilitation only to find out that he is not very much
different from when you started the program. He is not going to be a
very happy patient. Selection of the patient is extremely important in
reconstruction. There should be a good rapport between the doctor and
the patient. Each one should understand what the other is trying to do.

Why should it be done? The main reason is the patient's disability which
may be quite job related. One man we examined did not seem to me to
have very much actual disability, but after we talked further we discovered that he had been out of work eight to ten weeks every year for
the last five or six years because of his knee. This is sufficient indication to try to do something to improve his situation. Also, re-
creation is important. If a person is a tennis enthusiast and feels
that he has to play tennis, this is a different thing than if he is
not inclined toward athletic endeavors. So, it should be done if the
patient himself agrees that he needs to have something done.

When should it be done? If the doctor believes that he can do something
which will help, it should be done as quickly as the decision is made.
There is nothing to be gained by waiting another six months or longer
unless you are not sure this patient should have reconstruction. As
soon as you and the patient decide to do the reconstruction, you should
go ahead at that time with the necessary arrangements.

Where should it be done? It should be done some place equipped with staff,
instruments, and assistants to assure a workmanlike job. It should not
be done at a place where reconstruction is done once a month or twice
a year. I think it should be done in a hospital where this is more or

less a routine procedure. I would rate it much the same as I would for instrumentation of the spine, for example.

Who should do it? One must have some reservations here about who should do the operation. In the first place, it is an elective procedure and there is no urgency from the standpoint of time. Secondly, as this is in many cases a salvage procedure, a "last ditch" sort of thing, it should be done by someone who is well-versed in reconstruction techniques and who is doing them frequently. There is plenty of time to plan the procedure and develop the proper techniques to do it well. The surgeon who does one reconstruction a year probably doesn't do too good a job.

In our experimental operations on dogs, we have developed some ideas about tensile strength of various types of reconstruction [1-3]. In some instances the graft seemed to come up to almost a normal standard compared to the other leg. But the thing we more or less backed into, since we did not really start the experiments with that in mind, was the most important part of that particular project. Some of these dogs were kept as long as 5 years. We had a set-up where we took these dogs out in the country to a fenced-in enclosure where they could run. We paid the keeper on an increasing scale so that every month he kept the dog alive, he received a bigger fee. By the time 5 years had passed, he had a pretty good investment in those dogs, and he was really taking good care of them. We found almost without exception that the dogs which had an unstable knee, following our surgical procedures, had advanced arthritis. The dog 5 years postoperative with a stable knee had minimal or no arthritic changes. These findings are confirmed by the photographs of the appearance of the knees of the various dogs (Figs. 1, 2).

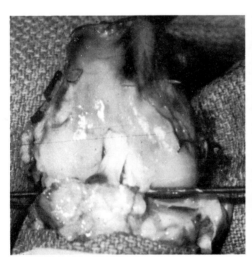
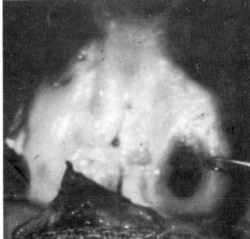

Fig. 1   Fig. 2

Fig. 1. Anterior cruciate reconstruction carried out in our experiments with dogs. Clinically and by gross specimen there was complete stability of the knee. Note femoral condyle shows no evidence of degenerative change [5]

Fig. 2. Dog sacrificed 4 1/2 years after repair of the anterior cruciate ligament. 3+ instability. Note extensive degenerative change when sacrificed at 4 1/2 years [5]

Incidence of arthritis in dogs

Grade of instability	Percent of arthritis
0-2+	14%
3-4+	80%

So, the dividend we got from that particular study is that there is
another indication for reconstruction; you not only do it for disability, but you do it to prevent advancing osteoarthritis in the joint.

Surgical Technique

The general plan of this medial collateral-posterior capsular reconstruction is that of advancement of the medial components distally on
the tibia and advancement of the posterior capsule distally on the
tibia. I do not strip out all the individual ligaments, but simply
take out the whole cuff of ligament from the midline in front to the
posteromedial border of the tibia, and back to the posterior midline.
This leaves the circulation and blood supply intact as the whole cuff
is pulled distally. This cuff may be of material that is very good,
or it may be quite weak. You can pretty well tell by looking at it if
it is going to be a suitable material for advancement.

With the patient supine, the leg is positioned at about 30° of flexion.
A bolster is placed beneath the thigh which should be well above the
popliteal space so that it does not press the popliteal structures
forward into the area of reconstruction.

The incision is medial parapatellar, beginning at about the central
portion of the patella and directly adjacent to it, extending through
the medial retinaculum distally along the medial edge of the patellar
tendon to the tibial tuberosity, at which point it swings posteromedially at approximately a 45° angle to the posteromedial border of the
tibia (Fig. 3). In reflecting this flap it is extremely important that

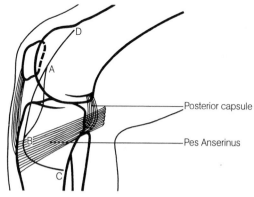

Posterior capsule

Pes Anserinus

Fig. 3. Lateral view of incisions used
for procedures on the medial side of
the knee: A to B for medial meniscectomy;
B to D for procedures on the patella;
and A to C for reconstruction of the
medial collateral ligament and posteromedial capsule [4]

all of the superficial tissue remains with the skin flap. That is, the
incision deepens immediately to the fascia, and the dissection is extended over the fascia. Thus, the superficial vessels and nerves are
in the flap and are cut at the site of the skin incision rather than
at the level of the posterior fold of the flap. This is the same in-

cision I ordinarily use for repair of acute injuries to the medial
side of the knee.

After the skin flap is developed back to the posterior margin of the
tibia, incision is made through the medial retinaculum extending along
the line of the skin incision to the top of the pes anserinus (Fig. 3).
The superior margin of the pes anserinus is quite definable through
the superficial fascia of the leg. This fascia is incised from the anterior border of the tibia directly along the top of the pes anserinus,
care being taken not to cut into the tendons in the pes itself. At
about midtibia the long fibers of the medial collateral ligament are
encountered. If the fascia and the ligament are adherent, no attempt
is made to separate them. The incision is carried right through the
long fibers at the level of the top of the pes. Usually in a reconstruction there has been a previous injury and previous incisions so that
the fascia and the long fibers of the medial collateral ligament may
be blended together. They should not be separated, but the incision
should be carried right through to the periosteum transecting the long
fibers at this level (Figs. 3, 4).

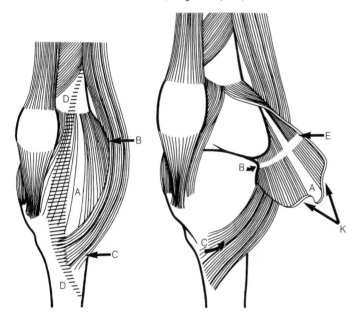

Fig. 4   Fig. 5

Fig. 4. Medial view of knee showing (crosshatched area D-D) the location of incision
through skin and subcutaneous tissue, (A) the long fibers of the medial collateral
ligament passing beneath (C) the pes anserinus, and (B) the posterior capsule underlying the hamstrings [4]

Fig. 5. Medial capsular and ligament flap reflected upward and backward after division of (A) the long fibers of the medial collateral ligament and (K) the fascia of
the leg along the upper edge of (C) the pes anserinus. Note that the length of the
flap decreases as incision proceeds posteriorly. At level of the midpoint of the
medial joint line the incision is 2 cm below joint line. Here the incision trans-
ects (E) the short capsular fibers of medial ligament. Further posteriorly the incision is only 1 cm below joint line where it divides (B) the tibial attachment of
the posterior capsule [4]

At this point the incision through the fascia follows the pes swinging proximally and posteriorly as the flap is reflected. The flap is removed from the tibia extraperiosteally and carried right up to the joint, where at about the midmedial point the short capsular fibers are encountered. These are divided at their tibial attachment just below the articular surface of the tibia. As the incision is extended posteriorly around the back of the tibia, the flap includes the fascia of the leg, the long fibers of the medial collateral ligament, the capsular layer of both medial collateral and posterior capsular components (Fig. 5). If the anterior extension of the semimembranosus is intimately bound to this flap, it is removed with the flap. If it is free, the dissection is carried around it. It is important to extend the detachment to the midline posteriorly. If the dissection is carried out right at the capsular attachment to the tibia, there is no risk of damage to the deep structures behind the knee. These structures drop backward since the flexed thigh is supported well above the knee. In order to get secure fixation posteriorly, the tibia is denuded subperiosteally with an elevator or, if necessary, with an osteotome so that there is raw bone from the posteromedial corner to the posterior midline. This does not reach the posterior cruciate ligament attachment, which is lower down on the tibia. By reflecting this flap, you achieve full access to the medial one-half of the top of the tibia. Any remnant of the medial meniscus is removed, and whatever intraarticular procedures are indicated are carried out, such as dissection of pannus off the medial femoral condyle, removal of osteocartilaginous foreign bodies, chondroplasty, etc.

Following this, the medial and posteromedial components are advanced downward and secured to the tibia by mattress sutures along its margin. The posterior capsular segment is reached by parallel drill holes using a 0.22 cm guide pin for a drill. This has the advantage of squeezing through the bone rather than grinding through it. Also, this pin will not break. Ordinarily, four holes are drilled from front to back beginning just at the medial edge of the patellar tendon about 2 cm below the top of the tibia, exiting at a similar point on the back of the tibia. Suitable protection is provided by an elevator or other instrument to prevent overpenetration of the pin into the popliteal space. Four, or sometimes five parallel holes are made entirely through the tibia. At about the same level, multiple drill holes (four to six) about 1 cm apart are made around the top of the tibia just through its cortex. The parallel holes are used for mattress sutures into the posterior

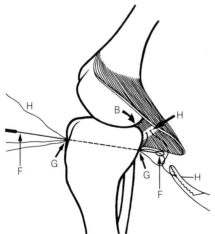

Fig. 6. Placement of (H) mattress sutures so as to advance (B) the posterior capsule downward on the tibia. (F) Ligature carrier carrying loop of suture has been passed from front to back through (GG) hole. The lateral limb of (H) the mattress suture has already been passed through tibia. The second limb is being passed through the ligature loop prior to pulling it and lateral limb of the next suture through the hole simultaneously. Four to five holes are used so that 3 or 4 mattress sutures are placed in the posterior capsule [4]

capsule (Fig. 6). With a suitable ligature carrier, a loop of suture
is passed from front to back through the most lateral hole. The loop
is pulled out into the wound posteriorly and a 1-0 cotton suture is
passed through the loop. We color code the sutures blue and white for
the posterior ones and white for the medial ones to avoid confusion.
After this first suture is sewn into the capsule, the loop is pulled
back through the second hole, and at the same time the first part of
the second mattress suture is pulled through this second hole. Usually
the capsular suture is at about the level of the bed of the excised
medial meniscus. This advances the capsule by a centimeter or two, the
exact amount being determined by the degree of relaxation of the posterior capsule.

Before the posterior sutures are completed, a row of superficial mattress sutures with 1-0 white cotton are passed through the holes around
the medial side of the tibia (Fig. 8). These sutures are placed at
this stage in order not to damage the through-and-through mattress
sutures since some of them will be in the same holes. These loops of
cotton are pulled through the drill holes in succession until all are
placed through the drill holes but not through the flap.

The posterior capsular sutures are then completed. At this point, traction on these mattress sutures should pull the posterior capsule snugly
against the back of the tibia (Fig. 7.H).

The medial mattress sutures are then sutured through the flap, positioned to advance the flap downward and forward as far as possible (Fig.
8). Usually this is at about the level of the meniscal bed, although
it does depend on the degree of relaxation which is present in any
particular patient. Tenacula are placed at the bottom of the flap. The
flap is oriented forward and downward as each separate mattress suture
is sewn through the entire flap, including the capsular ligament, the
long fibers of the medial collateral ligament, and the fascia, so that
the flap's anterior margin will reach the patellar tendon when all the
sutures are in place.

After these are all placed, the posterior capsular sutures are tied
(Fig. 8.H), first starting with the most lateral suture, moving in succession forward and medially. Thus, if any suture breaks, it can be
replaced without taking the whole flap down again.

After these posterior blue and white sutures are tightened and tied,
we continue from back to front tying the superficial mattress sutures.
One must be sure that the most forward edge of the flap will reach to
the patellar tendon. It is very easy to tether this flap too far backward in the placing of these mattress sutures. Instead, the tension
should be pulling the flap forward. While tension is maintained on the
flap with the tenacula, the white sutures are tied.

At this point the anterior attachment of the pes anserinus is detached
from the tibia by whatever amount is required to permit it to be pulled
up over the suture line of the distal portion of the flap. If the knee
has been quite relaxed, it may be necessary to remove the whole anterior
attachment. The distal edge of the flap which now contains the fascia
and the long fibers of the medial collateral ligament is sutured snugly
to the periosteum of the tibia and to the distal stump of the medial
collateral ligament, while the pes is retracted downward. Care should
be taken to secure the posterior edge of the flap to the underlying
tissue. The pes anserinus is then pulled up over the suture line and
securely sutured (Fig. 9). It is intended to weld this whole mass into
one homogeneous fibrous supporting structure.

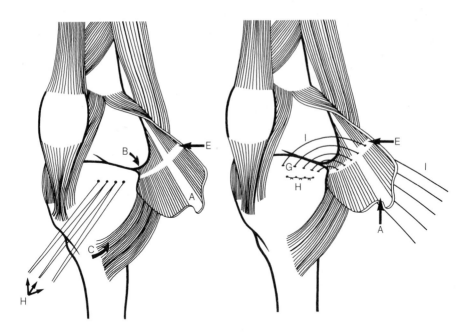

Fig. 7   Fig. 8

Fig. 7. The (H) mattress sutures have been placed, showing the anterior exit of
mattress sutures placed through the top of tibia and through the posterior capsule.
Traction on these sutures pulls (B) the capsule downward snugly against the tibia
at desired level. Usually the meniscal bed is well below the top of tibia, thus
shortening the capsule. This advancement is extended just to the posteromedial corner
but does not include (E) the short capsular fibers of medial collateral ligament.
(A) indicates the long fibers of the medial collateral ligament and (C) the pes anserinus [4]

Fig. 8. The (H) posterior capsular sutures tied and (I) the superficial mattress
sutures passed through (G) the holes in the cortex of the medial margin of the tibia.
The most posterior hole is placed well behind the posteromedial corner of tibia about
1 cm medial to the most medial posterior mattress suture. From 5 to 7 holes are made
progressing anteriorly. The medial mattress sutures (I) are passed through adjoining
holes and through full thickness of the flap (E) at a level providing the desired
flap tension.
(A) indicates long fibers of the medial collateral ligament [4]

Suction drainage is placed and the wound is closed. A long-leg posterior
plaster splint together with a lateral stirrup is applied rather than
a plaster cast. This permits variation in the size. It can be released
if the leg swells and can be tightened as the swelling goes down. It
can be removed if aspiration is necessary. After the leg stabilizes
in approximately 2 weeks, a long-leg plaster cast is applied with walking heel if the patient is quite active and has a relatively long muscular leg. This is worn for another 6 weeks, making a total of 8 weeks.
It is possible that at about 4 weeks a cast-brace be substituted for
the long-leg walking cast, since normal range of motion should not put
undue stress on the reconstruction.

The usual rehabilitative measures are carried out with instruction before and after surgery. Active exercises are conducted in the stirrup
splint and the cast: I have outlined a specific exercise program for

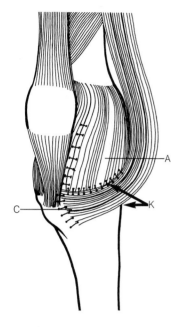

Fig. 9. Completed reconstruction. The pes anserinus has been detached from the tibia and reflected downward so that the entire ligament-capsular flap could be sutured to the periosteum and (A) stump of the long fibers of the medial collateral ligament beneath the pes. The (C) pes was then sutured over the flap. Note that (K) the fascia of the leg on the surface of flap now lies beneath the pes instead of overlying it as formerly (4)

the patient to follow. An example of the printed instructions I use is shown:

Rehabilative Exercises for the Lower Extremity
(O'Donoghue Orthopaedic Clinic)

Each of the following exercises should be done deliberately and to a particular count. In each one, raise the leg slowly to the count of three, hold it in the raised position to the count of three, lower it to the count of three and rest. Repeat this series ten times. Rest. Repeat the series ten more times, rest, and so on until a total of thirty series (three runs of ten) has been completed. The exercise should be repeated two or three times a day, depending upon your tolerance. Once you are able to complete this series of thirty, add weight and start a new series, adding weight gradually as your strength improves. Build this weight up to eleven kilograms if possible. Chart your daily progress and record it. Continue this until the involved thigh is (1) as large as the normal side, (2) as strong as the normal side, and (3) the range of knee motion is restored to normal.

The following exercises should be done as indicated previously:

1. Lying on the back, raise the leg up with the knee straight and not flexing.
2. Lie on the unaffected side. Raise the leg up with the knee straight.
3. Lie face down. Raise the leg up with the knee straight.
(N.B. In each instance, increase weight as previously indicated.)
4. Sitting with the leg hanging and the knee at a 90° angle, go through the series of exercises with spring resistance or weight on the foot. If there has been ligament damage or ligament reconstruction, a spring or system of pulleys and weights that resists extension of the knee is preferred to hanging the weight on the foot.
5. Lie face down with weight on the foot, flex the leg to vertical through the same series.

Exercises 1, 2, and 3 should be begun immediately postoperatively, or even started preoperatively. Exercises 4 and 5 should be done after removal of the cast and should not be done if there is swelling with effusion.

When the cast is removed, further rehabilitation continues according to the exigencies of the situation.

Results

The total number of reconstructions carried out by me at St. Anthony's Hospital, Oklahoma City, Oklahoma, between 1960 and 1970 was 335 [4]. Of these, 259 (77%) involved the medial side to a greater or lesser extent. 51 of this number (20%) had less than one year follow-up, so thus were not utilized in the survey. This leaves a total of 208 cases involving the medial side.

These 208 cases had reconstruction of the medial collateral ligament. However, as can be seen in Table 1, only 10% of these patients had reconstruction of the medial collateral alone. The medial side reconstruction I have described includes the medial side and posterior capsule. Sixty cases (30%) of the 208 would be included.

Table 1. Medial side with over one year follow-up

Medial side only	19	(10%)
Medial collateral and posterior capsule	41	(20%)
Medial collateral and anterior cruciate	20	(10%)
Medial collateral, posterior capsule, and anterior cruciate	53	(25%)
Other combinations of instability, such as posterior cruciate ligament, lateral collateral, or fibular collateral	75	(35%)
Number of cases	208	

This leaves 133 cases having medial side reconstruction involving some combination of the medial collateral, posterior capsule, and/or anterior cruciate. Table 2 gives a rating of improvement of stability. Those showing no significant improvement were rated 0. The remaining cases had from 1 to 4-Plus improvement, a 4-Plus improvement meaning that they had no demonstrable instability.

Table 2. Medial side reconstruction; 133 cases, excluding various combinations

Improvement in instability	
Degree	Medial
0	9
1+	50
2+	54
3+	17
4+	3

Complications

Complications were not excessive considering that most of the cases had had multiple operations before. However, as shown in Tables 3 and 4, there were specifically more complications in the cases which involved the anterior cruciate together with the medial and posterior capsule than those which involved the medial and posterior capsule alone

Table 3. Medial collateral or medial collateral and posterior capsule for 60 cases

Complications

Deep infection (healed)	1
Drainage (hematoma)	5
Synovitis (persistant)	2
Manipulation	1
Peroneal palsy (recovered)	1
Delayed flap healing	2

Table 4. Medial and anterior cruciate or medial and anterior cruciate and post. cap. for 73 cases

Complications

Deep infection (healed)	2
Drainage (hematoma)	13
Manipulation	3
Delayed flap healing	4
Re-operation	1
Thrombophlebitis (recovered)	2

Conclusion

I believe ligament reconstruction of the knee to be a worthwhile procedure. There was no case in this series which was actually worse after his operation [4]. Note that over half of the cases had better than 2-Plus improvement. Only 9 cases showed no significant improvement out of the 133 cases. I have emphasized the many variables which make each case an individual problem. Often the end result is not based entirely on stability and motion. There are socio-economic factors which may be extremely important. If the knee can be sufficiently tightened up so that a person can dispense with wearing a brace, cane, or crutches, to this person this represents a marked improvement even if actual examination of the knee might show considerable instability. It is extremely important to be wholly sympathetic with his physical and emotional problems. Some patients need marked stimulation in follow-up. Others need to be protected against overactivity. The fact that we are doing an increasing number of reconstructions each year is an indication of our overall satisfaction with the procedure.

References

1. O'DONOGHUE, D.H., ROCKWOOD, C.A., Jr., ZARICZNYJ, BASILIUS, KENYON, REX: Repair of knee ligaments in dogs. I. The lateral collateral ligament. J. Bone Joint Surg. 43A, 1167-1178 (Dec. 1961)
2. O'DONOGHUE, D.H., ROCKWOOD, C.A., Jr., FRANK, G.R., JACK, S.C., KENYON, REX: Repair of the anterior cruciate ligament in dogs. II. J. Bone Joint Surg. 48A, 503-519 (April 1966)
3. O'DONOGHUE, D.H., FRANK, G.R., JETER, G.L., JOHNSON, WILLIAM, ZEIDERS, J.W., KENYON, REX: Repair and reconstruction of the anterior cruciate ligament in dogs - Factors influencing long-term results. J. Bone Joint Surg. 53A, 710-718 (June 1971)
4. O'DONOGHUE, D.H.: Reconstruction for medial instability of the knee - Technique and results in sixty cases. J. Bone Joint Surg. 55A, 941-955 (July 1973a)
5. O'DONOGHUE, D.H.: The indications and surgical techniques of reconstruction for instability of the medical components of the knee. Jefferson Orthop. J. 2/1, 7-18 (1973)

9. Reconstruction of Chronic Medial Ligament Instability

S. L. James

Knee ligament surgery has its deepest roots in the work of PALMER, who published his remarkable report "On the Injuries to the Ligaments of the Knee Joint" in 1938. Unfortunately, his efforts were apparently upstaged by World War II, and serious ligament surgery laid relatively quiescent until the 1950s, when Dr. DON O'DONOGHUE stepped forth and presented the first of his data on acute knee ligament repair which opened the door to modern knee ligament surgery. Most of the early reconstructive surgeries were directed toward replacing specific anatomic structures, and on the medial side, the primary emphasis was on the superficial tibial collateral ligament with proximal or distal advancement, or tendon substitute. The track record was not particularly good, and knee ligament reconstructive surgery remained quite unpopular. With persistence of Dr. O'DONOGHUE and subsequently the contributions of SLOCUM, HUGHSTON, KENNEDY, NICHOLAS, and numerous others, significant improvements were made in the approach to chronic knee ligament reconstruction. About 1964 SLOCUM observed a rotational component on the medial side and described pathologic external tibial rotation in addition to valgus instability. KENNEDY was able to duplicate this type of instability in the laboratory, and in 1967 SLOCUM described the pes anserinus transplant designed to resist dynamically abnormal external tibial rotation and to provide reinforcement for other reconstructive procedures used to stabilize the medial side of the knee.

Currently, knee ligament instabilities are classified as "One-plane" and "rotational" based upon abnormal motion of the tibia in relation to the femoral condyles. One-plane instabilities are in the sagittal and coronal planes, manifested by a positive anterior or posterior drawer sign in the sagittal plane and valgus or varus instability in the coronal plane. Rotational instabilities are classified by the presence of abnormal rotation of the tibial plateaus in relation to the femoral condyles. The rotational instabilities are anteromedial, posteromedial, anterolateral and posterolateral. Anteromedial rotational instability refers to abnormal tibial rotation with the medial tibial plateau subluxing anteriorly and rotating externally. This discussion concerns the combination of valgus and anteromedial rotatory instability.

The initial injury is one of valgus stress and excessive external tibial rotation. Typically a blow to the posterolateral aspect of the knee, forcing it into valgus and externally rotating the femur on a fixed tibia, results in sequential injury to the deep capsular ligament, postero-oblique ligament, superficial tibial collateral ligament, anterior cruciate ligament and perhaps the medial one-half of the posterior capsule. The extent of injury to these structures may vary from case to case depending upon the magnitude and direction of the forces applied as well as the relative position of the femur and tibia and the amount of displacement and dynamic forces exerted by muscles at the time of injury.

Diagnosis of Instability

Clinically, patients with this type of instability typically complain
of giving way with a change in direction. Running straight ahead is
often no problem, but sudden cutting, pivoting or twisting on the involved extremity creates instability. The diagnosis is generally quite
straight forward and is done by performing the abduction stress test
and the Slocum test for rotatory instability.

The abduction stress test is performed initially with the knee in full
extension, and then with 30° of flexion. One-plane valgus instability
with the knee in full extension indicates very serious ligamentous
laxity implicating the medial ligaments, the medial one-half of the
posterior capsule, the anterior cruciate ligament, and perhaps the
posterior cruciate ligament. The posterior cruciate ligament, however,
will be involved only if there has been severe subluxation or dislocation. Certainly, if the test is positive with the knee in full extension, it will also be positive at 30° of flexion. If the abduction
stress test is negative in full extension, it indicates that the posterior capsule and posterior cruciate ligaments are intact. The knee
is then flexed to 30° and stressed again. This relaxes the posterior
capsule, removing its stabilizing effect and any medial ligamentous
laxity will be manifested by medial joint space-opening. It is interesting to note that there is usually some associated rotational instability with the abduction stress test, and if the leg is held internally rotated, the amount of valgus instability is less than if the
leg is allowed to rotate externally. The explanation for this is that
with an intact posterior cruciate, external rotation relaxes the ligament allowing more medial opening of the joint, while internal rotation tightens the posterior cruciate which holds the medial condyle
and plateau in closer approximation.

The rotatory instability test is performed with the patient lying re-
layed in a supine position, the hip flexed 45°, the knee flexed 90°,
and the foot secured by the examiner sitting across the forefoot. The
proximal calf is grasped with both hands and pulled forward. The tibia
is observed for abnormal motion in relation to the femoral condyles.
This test is performed with the foot in three positions. Initially,
the foot is placed in 30° of internal rotation, the 15° of external
rotation, and then finally in neutral position. The test is negative
with internal rotation when the lateral ligaments and posterior cruciate
ligaments are intact. Repeating the test with the foot and leg externally rotated, stresses the medial ligaments and the anterior cruciate
ligament. If these structures are lax, the medial tibial plateau will
sublux anteriorly and rotate laterally in relation to the medial femoral condyle. The amount of instability increases with serial rupture
of the deep capsular ligament, the superficial tibial collateral ligament, posterior oblique ligament, and the anterior cruciate ligament.
If these structures are mildly injured, the test may not be positive
because the posterior horn of the medial meniscus can block the forward
movement and external rotation of the tibial plateau; however, usually
there is some mild rotatory instability present, and one can suspect
this situation from the history of a significant injury and more functional deficit than is usually found with simply a meniscal injury.
The test is finally repeated with the tibia and foot in neutral position. A positive test indictes the anterior cruciate ligament to some
extent. A significant anterior subluxation of both tibial plateaus in
this position indicates additional laxity of both the medial and lateral
structures, a complex form of ligament instability.

In addition to determining medial ligament stability, patellar stability should also be investigated. If the anteromedial retinaculum was also injured, it may have healed in a relaxed fashion, creating lateral patellar instability. This will also have to be taken into consideration when planning reconstructive surgery.

Once the diagnosis of chronic medial instability has been made, the degree of functional deficit must be determined before a decision on surgical reconstruction is made. A mild degree of instability may be stabilized by appropriate muscle rehabilitation, but the final decision is dependent upon how much limitation is created for the patient. Ligament reconstruction is a serious undertaking and must be thoroughly explained to the patient. Some individuals may desire simply to modify their activity a little rather than undergo surgery. Once surgery has been selected, the surgeon must be fully aware of the pathological variations he may encounter and the various reconstructive procedure which may be required. A technically perfect procedure inappropriately applied is destined to failure.

Reconstruction Method

The procedure to be described was developed predominantly by Dr. DON SLOCUM.

Surgery is performed with the patient lying supine, the knee flexed to $90°$ or more over the end of the table and the thigh supported by a triangular bolster placed proximally well clear of the popliteal area. An incicion is made starting proximally at the medial femoral epicondyle, coursing distally along the inferior margin of the vastus medialis obliquus, then curving distally to parallel the medial border of the patellar tendon and then terminating distal to the tibial tubercle at the lower border of the pes anserinus (Fig. 1A and B). A skin flap including subcutaneous fat is developed posteriorly to expose the entire medial aspect of the knee from the patellar tendon anteriorly to the popliteal space posteriorly. The incision appears curved with knee flexed but is almost straight when the knee is extended.

The knee is re-examined and areas of ligamentous laxity identified, confirming the preoperative findings and perhaps noting additional instability not readily apparent without an anesthetic. An anteromedial incision is made through the retinaculum and capsule, and the joint thoroughly inspected. The incision is placed more laterally, directly along the medial edge of the patellar tendon if the anteromedial retinaculum has been attenuated and the patella is unstable. This facilitates later reconstruction of the anteromedial retinaculum. Inspect the articular cartilages, menisci, and the cruciate ligaments. Remember that the mere presence of the cruciate ligaments does not indicate their functional capacity. Interstitial damage may have rendered the ligaments partially or totally incompetent in spite of their grossly normal appearance. Medial meniscectomy is routinely performed in reconstruction, and the anterior one-half of the meniscus is easily released through this incision. Frequently, posterior horn tears are encountered from attrition, but even without a definite tear, meniscectomy facilitates mobilization of the medial capsule necessary for reconstruction. After the meniscectomy, again check for anteromedial rotatory instability. It will often be even more apparent once the stabilizing effect of the posterior horn has been removed.

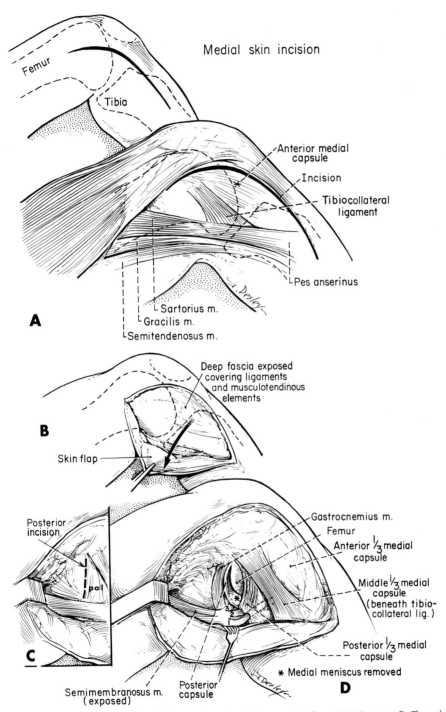

Medial skin incision

A
- Femur
- Tibia
- Anterior medial capsule
- Incision
- Tibiocollateral ligament
- Pes anserinus
- Sartorius m.
- Gracilis m.
- Semitendenosus m.

B
- Deep fascia exposed covering ligaments and musculotendinous elements
- Skin flap

C
- Posterior incision
- pol
- Semimembranosus m. (exposed)
- Posterior capsule

D
- Gastrocnemius m.
- Femur
- Anterior ⅓ medial capsule
- Middle ⅓ medial capsule (beneath tibio- collateral lig.)
- Posterior ⅓ medial capsule
- * Medial meniscus removed

Fig. 1. A The medial incision and underlying anatomic structures. B The skin flap is reflected postiorly, exposing the entire medial side of the knee. C An incision is made along the posterior margin of the posterior oblique ligament (pol) to expose the posterior joint. D The completed postior medial exposure. Three heads of semimembranosus are shown: (1) the anteromedial head, (2) the direct head, and (3) the oblique popliteal ligament

Attention is next directed to the posterior medial aspect of the knee where the deep fascia is incised vertically from the adductor tubercle to the upper border of the sartorius. Fatty tissue is dissected away to expose the semimembranosus tendon, the medial head of the gastrocnemius, the posterior one-third of the medial capsule, and the medial portion of the posterior capsule. The knee is again stressed and areas of laxity noted. Next, identify the relatively nonyielding, thick portion of the posterior one-third of the medial capsule lying posterior to the superficial tibial collateral ligament and oriented obliquely from above downward and posteriorly. This is a portion of the posterior oblique ligament and is a key to stabilizing the posterior medial aspect of the knee. Even with the knee acutely flexed, this element is not as redundant as the thinner, more posterior part of the medial capsule which blends with the posterior capsule forming a sling about the medial femoral condyle. An oblique incision is made along the trailing edge of this ligamentous thickening (Fig. 1C). The incision starts at the epicondylar level and terminates at the tibial insertion near the direct head of the semimembranosus tendon which inserts onto the posterior tibial tubercle. Proper placement of the incision allows ready access to the posterior medial compartment of the knee. If necessary, the remainder of the medial meniscus can be removed very readily through this incision (Fig. 1D).

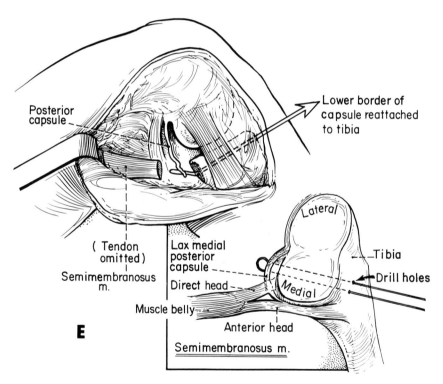

Fig. 1E-G. Repair of the medial half of the posterior capsule by reattaching to a freshened bony bed with sutures passed through the proximal tibia

At this point, the reconstruction is ready to commence. If the medial one-half of the posterior capsule is lax, it must be reattached to the posterior margin of the medial tibial plateau (Fig. 1E-F). A new bed is prepared with an osteotome immediately below the articular margin.

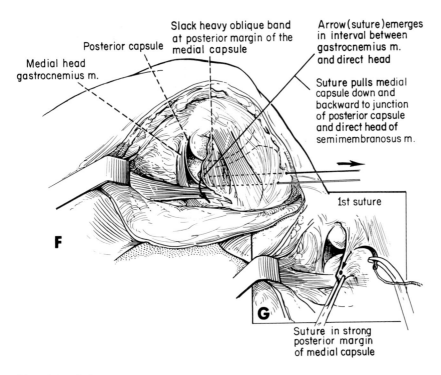

Medial head
gastrocnemius m.

Posterior capsule

Slack heavy oblique band
at posterior margin of the
medial capsule

Arrow(suture)emerges
in interval between
gastrocnemius m.
and direct head

Suture pulls medial
capsule down and
backward to junction
of posterior capsule
and direct head of
semimembranosus m.

1st suture

F

G

Suture in strong
posterior margin
of medial capsule

Fig. 1F and G

Three drill holes are made from anterior to posterior through the proximal tibia exiting in the prepared bed posteriorly. Three heavy sutures
are placed in the posterior capsule at the level of the former meniscal
attachment. These sutures are pulled through the drill holes with a
ligature passer and tied anteriorly securing the posterior capsule to
its new bed. The posterior capsule should now be snug with extension.

The next step is to tighten the posterior one-third of the medial capsule (Fig. 1F and G), but remember to close the anteromedial incision
first. Two to three heavy mattress sutures are placed in the posterior
inferior portion of the posterior oblique ligament previously described
(Fig. 2). The first suture is placed at the level of the joint, and the
next suture immediately above. They are passed distally and posteriorly
through the medial edge of the posterior capsule and then through the
direct head of the semimembranosus. An attempt should be made to keep
these sutures extrasynovial if possible. The sutures are then pulled
tight and tied. This serves to pull the posterior oblique ligament
downward and postiorly, and tenses the oblique popliteal ligament posteriorly which is an expansion of the semimembranosus. More proximally
the incision is closed by imbricating the medial edge of the posterior
capsule over the redundant posterior medial capsule completing the reefing procedure.

The semimembranosus tendon is brought up and forward where it is secured
over the repair without releasing its direct head. Then the medial head
is released from its insertion under the superficial tibial collateral
ligament, brought proximally and anteriorly, and sutured over the superficial tibial collateral for additional dynamic and static reinforcement
to the repair. Be certain these sutures pass only through the super-

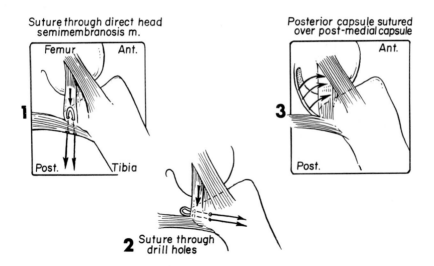

Fig. 2. 1 The posterior medial capsule (posterior oblique ligament) is tightened by pulling it posteriorly and distally, securing it to the direct head of the semimembranosus tendon. 2 If the direct head is inadequate, the sutures may be placed through drill holes. 3 The repair is completed proximally by drawing the medial half of the posterior capsule forward and imbricating it over the trailing border of the posterior oblique ligament

ficial tibial collateral and not into the deep capsular ligament, or they will restrict the normal gliding motion of the superficial tibial collateral.

In the event that the anteromedial retinaculum is lax, and there is associated patellar instability, a medial one-half patellar tendon transplant and anteromedial retinacular reefing is done (Fig. 3A and B). This, however, must be accomplished before the posterior medial reconstruction is completed. If not, it is virtually impossible to close the anteromedial incision. The medial one-third to one-half of the patellar tendon is split longitudinally and released distally from the tibial tubercle. The anteromedial retinaculum is then advanced anteriorly and secured to the remaining free edge of the patellar tendon, removing any laxity anteromedially. It is best initially to place the sutures proximally near the distal pole of the patella and work distally to facilitate the closure. The medial one-half of the patellar tendon is pulled distally, transferred about 2 cm posteriorly, and secured to the proximal tibia under a periosteal bridge. This further reinforces the retinaculum and also serves to help stabilize the patella.

Should the anteromedial retinaculum be stretched to the point that the vastus medialis obliquus has migrated proximally, this muscle may be mobilized and advanced distally over the anteromedial retinaculum taking care not to advance it past the midportion of the patella. Leaving a 5 mm cuff of retinaculum about the margin of the vastus medialis obliquus facilitates suturing it into its new position. This further reinforces the anteromedial retinaculum dynamically and also helps stabilize the patella.

The final step is the pes anserinus transfer to reinforce dynamically the static ligament reconstruction. The lower border of the pes anserinus is identified, making certain to include the semitendinosus. Care should also be taken to identify the sartorial branch of the sa-

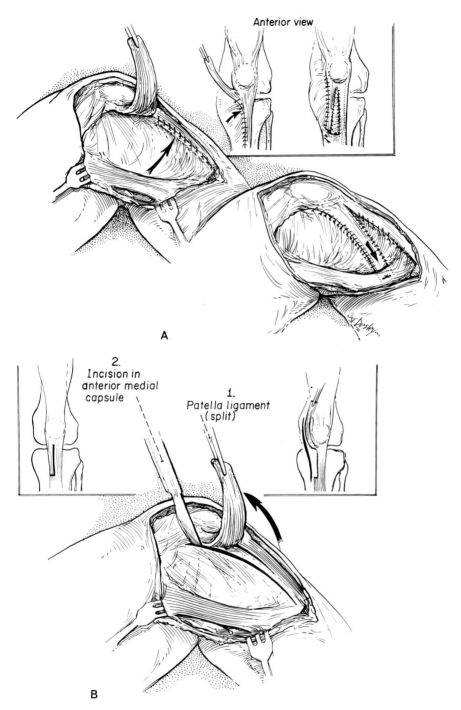

Anterior view

2.
Incision in
anterior medial
capsule

1.
Patella ligament
(split)

A

B

Fig. 3A and B. The medial half of the patellar tendon transplant and anteromedial
retinacular reefing

phenous nerve which exits between the sartorius and the gracilis at about the musculotendinous junction of the sartorius and then courses distally into the subcutaneous tissue. After the lower border of the pes anserinus has been identified, it is freed and the lower two-thirds of the conjoined tendon including the semitendinosus and gracilis is released from the tibia. This portion of the pes anserinus is then folded proximally upon itself, bringing the semitendinosus and gracilis under the flare of the tibia. Do not bring it to joint line level. The lower border of the semitendinosus is freed proximally just far enough to allow the transfer to be accomplished easily. If dissection is carried too far proximally, the semitendinosus will sublux over the medial femoral condyle as the knee is extended. The released portion of the pes anserinus is advanced anteriorly and secured along the medial margin of the tibial tubercle and distal portion of the patellar tendon with heavy 1-O suture. Place the sutures so that the ends are located on the medial side of the tibial tubercle and patellar tendon and will not create nuisance protuberances subcutaneously. The most common mistake in performing the pes anserinus transplant is not to include the semitendinosus and either to cut or place the sartorial branch of the saphenous nerve under tension.

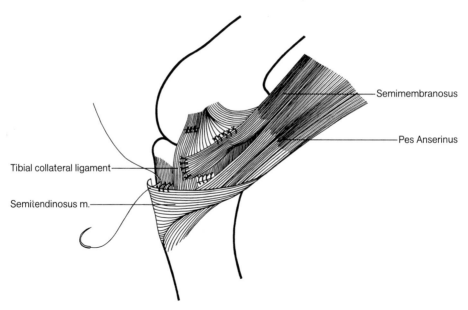

Fig. 4. Pes anserinus transplant. The lower 1/2 to 2/3 of the pes anserinus including the semitendinosus tendon and the gracilis tendons have been reflected proximally on the tibia and sutured into position along the medial border of the tibial tubercle and distal portion of the patellar ligament, thus creating a sling under the medial flare of the tibia. This enhances the internal rotatory effect of the semitendinosus tendon, which now becomes the more proximal structure of the pes anserinus. Also depicted are release and proximal transfer of the medial limb of the semimembranosus tendon, attaching it to the midlateral capsule and ligamentous structures of the knee to provide further dynamic support. More proximally, the direct tendon of the semimembranosus has been reefed into the posteromedial capsular repair

The pes anserinus transfer may be modified to provide additional reinforcement for a severely attenuated midmedial capsule and tibial collateral ligament. In this situation, the sartorius is left attached distally and mobilized proximally along its superior and inferior margin. It is then secured obliquely across the midmedial joint line and along the lower margin of the vastus medialis obliquus. The gracilis and semitendinosus are transferred in the usual fashion (Fig. 5). The effectiveness of the pes anserinus transplant with this procedure is probably changed very little in view of the fact that semitendinosus is the most effective internal tibial rotator after the transfer.

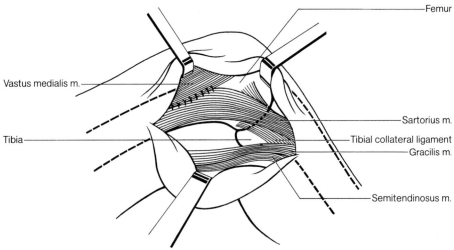

Fig. 5. Modification of the pes anserinus transfer in which the sartorius muscle is .disected free from proximal to distal leaving it attached at its distal insertion. The muscle is relocated obliquely across the midportion of the joint and sutured · along the trailing edge of the vastus medialis muscle. This creates a dynamic reinforcement for attenuated medial structures. The gracilis and semitendinosus tendons are transfered in their usual fashion to function as the pes anserinus plasty

Upon completing reconstruction, the tourniquet is released and hemostasis achieved. The wound is closed with a large suction tube left under the medial flap. Dressings and a long-leg cast are applied with the knee flexed 45°-50°. The tibia is slightly internally rotated. The cast is often changed at 3 or 4 days to insure a snug fit and again at 2 weeks when the sutures are removed. Total plaster immobilization is 8 weeks. The last 3 weeks are in a hinged cylinder cast which allows motion between 30° and 60°. Following removal of the cast, a derotation knee brace, the Lenox Hill Brace, is worn full time for an additional 4 months. Rehabilitation is best accomplished under the direct supervision of a registered physical therapist. Emphasis is not placed upon early return of full range of motion for fear of stretching out the repair. Initially, the program consists of gentle range of motion exercise and isometrics. With the return of muscle tone and control, progressive resistive exercises are included. Be certain that all muscles from the hip distally are included. Too often only the quadriceps are emphasized. The goal is restoration of bulk, strength and endurance of all lower extremity muscles. Eventually the program progresses to more functional endeavor involving controlled maneuvers while running. A period of some 8-12 months will be required for adequate ligament healing and muscle rehabilitation.

Suggested Reading

1. SLOCUM, D.B., LARSON, R.L.: J.Bone Joint Surg. 50A, 211 (1968)
2. HUGHSTON, J.C. et al.: J. Bone Joint Surg. 58A, 159, 173-179 (1976)

3. KENNEDY, J.C.: Classification of knee ligament instabilities. Report to American Orthopedic Society for Sports Medicine, Committee on Research and Education, 1976
4. KENNEDY, J.C. et al.: J. Bone Joint Surg. 56A, 223 (1974)
5. KENNEDY, J.C. et al.: J. Bone Joint Surg. 58A, 350 (1976)
6. NOYES, F.R. et al.: J. Bone Joint Surg. 56A, 1406 (1974)
7. NOYES, F.R., GROOD, E.S.: J. Bone Joint Surg. 58A, 1074 (1976)
8. WARREN, L.F. et al.: J. Bone Joint Surg. 56A, 665 (1974)
9. SLOCUM, D.B. et al.: J. Sports Med. 2, 123 (1974)
10. HUGHSTON, J.C., EILERS, A.F.: J. Bone Joint Surg. 55A, 923 (1973)
11. O'DONOGHUE, D.H.: J. Bone Joint Surg. 32A, 721 (1950)
12. O'DONOGHUE, D.H.: J. Bone Joint Surg. 55A, 941 (1973)
13. PALMER, I.: Acta Chir. Scand. (Suppl. 53) 81, 3 (1938)
14. FOX, J.M. et al.: Am. J. Sports Med. 4, 131 (1976)
15. NOYES, F.R., SONSTEGARD, D.A.: Biomechanical function of the pes anserinus at the knee and effect of its transplantation on rotatory instability. In: Proceedings of the Annual Meeting of the Orthopaedic Research Society, Washington, D.C., 1972
16. SLOCUM, D.B., LARSON, R.L.: J. Bone Joint Surg. 50A, 226 (1958)
17. BAUMGARTL, F.: Das Kniegelenk. Berlin-Göttingen-Heidelberg: Springer, 1964, p. 153
18. SLOCUM, D.B. et al.: Clin. Orthop. 100, 23 (1974)
19. ERIKSSON, E.: Med. Science in Sports 8, 133 (1976)
20. JAMES, S.L. et al.: Prosthetic cruciate ligaments in reconstruction of the unstable knee - A preliminary peear review. Presented at the 44th Annual Meeting of the American Academy of Orthopedic Surgeons, Las Vegas, Feb. 1977
21. GALWAY, R.D. et al.: J. Bone Joint Surg. 54B, 763 (1972)
22. CABAUD, H.E., SLOCUM, D.B.: Am. J. Sports Med. 5, No. 3 (1977)
23. JAMES, S.L.: Instructional course. American Academy of Orthopedic Surgeons, Las Vegas, Feb. 1977
24. ELLISON, A.E.: In paper presented to American Orthopedic Society for Sports Medicine, New Orleans, 1975
25. SLOCUM, D.B.: Personal communication
26. NICHOLAS, J.A.: J. Bone Joint Surg. 55A, 899 (1973)

Discussion

PUHL: What type of derotation brace do you advise?

JAMES: We use the Lenox Hill derotation brace. I think this is presently the most effective brace for anteromedial rotatory instability. I feel that following removal of the cast, the ligaments should still be protected for quite some time. We know that it requires much longer than 8 weeks for ligaments to mature. We also know that motion allows them to mature more rapidly; the collagen fibrils are also reorientated more rapidly, and the intermolecular bonding occurs more readily. However, I still feel that the patient should be protected during a certain period to prevent reinjuries. I think the derotation brace will allow an adequate amount of activity and a maximum of protection.

PARSCH: Dr. JAMES, what chances would you give competitive athletes of returning to their sports after a one-year interruption?

JAMES: I think anyone who has required an extensive procedure such as this for reconstruction should not plan on going back to a contact type of sport. In particular, I usually advise such patients not to reconsider footfall or wrestling, i.e., sports where there is a high incidence of knee ligament injury. Hopefully they would be able to return to some of the less vigorous types of sports, such as tennis or perhaps racket ball. We even have people skiing; of course, there is a higher risk of injury there, but I often also ask these patients to wear the derotation brace during periods of heavy physical activity.

THIEL: Dr. JAMES, are your patients allowed swimming and cycling during the time in which your patients are wearing this derotation brace?

JAMES: Yes, swimming and cycling are an integral part of their rehabilitation program. Of course they need not wear the brace during that type of activity.

THIEL: They do not need it when they are swimming?

JAMES: No. I think in swimming the knee is quite well protected and the body is buoyed up by the water. I would not advise them to do the breast stroke with that kind of kick, but the crawl would be all right.

KARPF: Do you treat the cruciate ligament when you have an anteromedial ligament instability? If not, does this not in time result in an instability?

JAMES: Initially we did not treat these anterior cruciate ligaments, but for the past few years I have been using the Eriksson procedure for very severe instabilities. I think this is a good point. We used to think we could avoid repair of the anterior cruciate ligament, and I think we perhaps can in milder cases if we use the pes anserinus and other types of muscular reinforcement. However, for this severe type of instability with a very significant anterior displacement of the tibia, I think we have to develop some means of replacing or substituting for the anterior cruciate ligament.

COTTA: Dr. JAMES, do you have any long-term follow-ups of this method, and what are the statistics concerning osteoarthritis?

JAMES: We hope that by stabilizing a knee statically or dynamically we can avoid a lot of the abnormal motion which would lead to osteoarthrosis. As I stated, this procedure evolved over a period of years and finally reached this point of development in about the last 4 to 5 years. We have not done a long-term follow-up of these; we plan to have this accomplished during the next year. My impression is that although these people retain some element of static instability, they do quite well functionally. I think it is the muscular reinforcement that is providing adequate dynamic stability. Only time will tell whether or not this type of procedure is actually preventing the development of osteoarthrosis.

JAKOB: We have seen that with the Don 2 procedure the distal attachment of the medial collateral ligament is routinely taken off and advanced distally and anteriorly. How do you procede?

JAMES: We do not routinely take off the tibial collateral ligament or the superficial collateral ligament if it has healed in position. We feel that removing this can be accomplished adequately posteriorly or anteriorly.

JAKOB: If, however, there is instability, do you take it off?

JAMES: If necessary we will, and advance it.

WEBER: Dr. O'DONOGHUE, would you operate a housewife with the same procedures, or would you say that these operations are in general for athletes only?

O'DONOGHUE: No I do not think that this is for athletes only. As a matter of fact, Dr. JAMES stated he does not usually advise an athlete to return to contact sport. I think that a housewife is just as desirous of a stable knee as any male. We have a lot of E.R.A. in our country where the woman wants equality.

COTTA: Up to which age would you perform this reconstructive operation on the knee joint?

O'DONOGHUE: We ought to have an operation limit, but I have noticed that as you grow older, you more readily want to take someone of your own age; I recognize that I would not like to have an unstable knee myself and I can see how somebody else at may age might not either.

WEBER: Dr. JAMES, did you ever see unstable knee joints of the medial collateral type in children? These injuries are quite frequent in down-hill skiing of children. I have never seen a late instability in a child. Could you explain this phenomenon?

JAMES: I agree with you; I havn't either. Again, I think that the growth potential of the child is working in our favor and that consequently with additional growth, the ligamentous structures have the capacity of again becoming snug. The adult has lost this capability.

KRAHL: Dr. O'DONOGHUE, when does the "early reconstruction" end and when does the "late reconstruction" begin?

O'DONOGHUE: I think the question is: When can you do an acute ligament repair, and when do you have to do reconstruction. We said that an acute ligament repair should be done within 2 weeks after injury. After this point, i.e., from 2 until 8 or 10 weeks (and in some cases as late as 12 weeks), it is probably not advisable to operate. If, however, at the end of this time the knee is still unstable, then a reconstruction would be possible. In some cases a reconstruction could already be done after 8 weeks.

There are exceptions to that. In particular, if you have decided to repair an anterior cruciate, you should do it as soon as possible, the reason for this being that the retraction of the torn cruciate liga-ment can change the repair from a quite simple matter which it usually is into a very difficult undertaking. We certainly attempt to do this repair within 2 weeks.

To illustrate this with an example, suppose you have an abraison of the skin which is now 2 or 3 days old, I think the danger of infection would override the urgency of an immediate operation of the anterior cruciate. In such a case, I have operated as late as 3 or 4 weeks. Then it is a very difficult job, because at this time healing has oc-curred, the blood has coagulated, and it is very difficult to define the pathology.

Sometimes when you try to determine where the tear is, you may actually do more damage to the ligament. I think you should do a repair within a week, 10 days, or 2 weeks. One day will be better than one week.

JAMES: I agree with this philosophy! I think that if surgery is delayed for one or the other reason beyond the 2 to 3 weeks, particularly be-yond 2 weeks, you may as well just wait and see what is going to happen to this knee. It may be one of these that will heal adequately with conservative treatment. Very often when I see a patient late after a knee injury, I will start immediately with the rehabilitation phase and see whether or not the patient actually is going to develop a func-tional deficit which limits his activity significantly.

MOSCHI: I do have some criticism that I would like to make concerning the type of surgery that has just now been presented. I can explain it best by referring to the biomechanics of the knee. The evolute of the knee joint, studied by FICK, is within the condyle profile, and that is on the femoral side of the knee joint. The instant centers of rotation are within the femoral side of the knee joint. What does this mean? It means that nature "built" the ligaments of the knee joint in such a way that they are concentric into the femoral condyles. Both the middle third and the posterior third of the capsular ligament are included. So, whenever we do any surgical repair on these ligaments, it is just in the opposite way that nature built those ligaments. We are doing something that may not be so satisfactory, except in one case which I shall explain afterwards. When we see the instant centers of rotation of both femoral condyles, we notice that both slopes stay in the femoral part of the joint, although they both describe different curves. What is very important at this moment are the menisci. The menisci are not there just for static purposes; they are there for dynamic purposes. We know that an extramural meniscectomy - a meniscectomy performed as Professor TRILLAT suggests - does not effect the knee joint. But in the case of an O'Donoghue knee reconstruction, we are not performing an extramural, but an intramural meniscectomy, and therefore we are certainly taking a stabilizing element out of the joint. Dr. JAMES showed us some meniscus degeneration which was due to incongruency of the joint but occurred after a certain delay.

If we have to perform surgery on knee ligaments for a medial reconstruction, except in the case where the original injury involved a part of the ligaments situated between the meniscus and the tibia, I do not see why we should do an O'Donoghue reconstruction for other ligamentous injuries. I would say that over 60% of these injuries concern part of the ligament situated between the menisci and the condyles. Anyone with experience with acute injuries knows that most of the pathology in the injuries is above the level of the menisci. If so, I do not see why we should take the ligaments off the tibia and bring them down to the tibia again. I have two main reasons. First of all, we are going to be dealing with scar tissue because the reconstruction of that ligament is done with connective tissue and not with the strong, thick, dense tissue of a ligament. Secondly, we are not going to help the biomechanics by taking out the mensici.

Dr. JAMES and Dr. O'DONOGHUE showed and told us several times that the most important part of knee reconstruction is the vascularization of the ligaments. Therefore we must encourage the revascularization of the muscles and the ligaments the best way we can after our reconstructions.

We know that the ligaments in the middle part of the knee are not passive structures. They are not only there for avoiding detraction of the joint; when the semimembranosus is in contraction, it bends the fibers of the ligaments so that the ligaments apply compression to the joint. Therefore the medial compartment ligaments are active stabilizers of the knee. In order to be good active stabilizers they also need the presence of the meniscus or at least the mural part of the meniscus.

What we want to point out with this biomechanic simplification of the action of the ligament of the medial compartment is that the most important part of the ligament is the one above the layer of the meniscus. Seen biomechanically, if anything must be done to reinforce the structures, it is to bring up this part of the meniscus, not down. The mural part of the mensicus must be lifted towards the epicondyle and the adaptor's tubercles using any method we know. Therefore, excluding the lesions of ligaments underneath the meniscus level, the best biomechanic results for all other lesions can be achieved when the reconstruction is performed in such a way as to bring the ligaments up towards the epicondyle at the adductor's tubercle. It is not my purpose to present that surgery, since it has been published in the Bone and Joint Surgery Journal by Dr. HUGHSTON and his team.

I have a little criticism on the pes anserinus transplant. The first two or three times that I performed the pes anserinus transplant it did not work satisfactorily I was probably removing the saphenous nerve during the surgery. However, I was also doing something else that was not satisfactory for the patients. After having read the NOYES paper in the Journal of Bone and Joint Surgery, I agree completely with his statement that the semitendinosus is the muscle which most reinforces the internal rotation. This means that the semitendinosus is the most active internal rotator in the pes transplant; therefore I avoid doing a complete Slocum procedure which requires cutting off the distal insertion of the pes anserinus. From transplanting only the semitendinosus we know from hand surgery on polio patients that whenever we cut off the insertion of a tendon, we are going to lose some of the function of the tendon. Therefore, instead of taking out all the distal insertion of the pes anserinus, I just take the tendon of the semitendinosus and bring it forward and upward about 2-3 cm. I put some nonabsorbable stitches close to the distal insertion of the patella tendon. In my opinion this gives me an active reinforcement of the internal rotation without destroying the distal insertion of the same tendon. In my opinion it is very important that the bursa is between the pes anserinus and the tibia, because if we have a hematoma in the bursa, we are going to have some scar tissue at that level, implying the loss of the biomechanical part of the pes anserinus transplant.

I would like to ask Dr. JAMES for his opinion in this modification, for which, by the way, I do not claim sole authorship. I would also like to ask Dr. O'DONOGHUE if he feels that the biomechanic basis of his reconstruction of the knee ligaments does give the knee as much biomechanic support as possible, although I agree that in his hands his surgery is having excellent results.

I would like to say one more thing with regards to postoperative care. I saw that both of you were presenting a straight-leg cast or a mildly flexed cast. We know from BOUSQUET'S work of 1964/1965, I suppose, that the most instable positions of the knee is at 60^{0}-90^{0}. If we want the ligaments to be as tight as possible, we should put the knee at 60^{0} of flexion because that is the only position where the middle compartment ligaments are completely relaxed. If I do a reconstruction I want to have my ligaments as tight as possible; afterwards I am going to stretch them in the same way you said. In my hands that requires 6-8 months.

JAMES: I think you are fooling yourself if you think you can restore the instant center of rotation accurately where most of the lesions do occur above the meniscus. Research has been done that shows that if you tamper with the more proximal portion of the tibial collateral ligament, you are quite likely going to disturb the instant centers of rotation more than if you work distally. You can do almost anything you want to with the superficial tibial collateral ligament, moving it distally, and still not disturb the instant centers of rotation. I think that when you are dealing with scar tissue, the anatomy is at best very difficult to recognize. When you say that you can restore the instant center accurately by repositioning proximally, you are trying to achieve something that is very difficult to accomplish consistently. We are dealing with a structure that has been badly damaged. You may be able to do this in a specimen where the anatomy is quite normal, but since this is not always the case, I would prefer to work more distally than proximally. As for the pes anserinus transfer modification, I think the important thing about the pes anserinus is its principle, not necessarily the way that it is conducted. Over a 14-year period now we have not had any serious problems with the pes anserinus as long as it is carried out properly, and, as I pointed out, the semitendinosus portion is the important part; the way that this is accomplished is not so important as the principle behind it. As far as mobilisation following surgery is concerned, the slide I showed did not have the knee flexed as much as we normally do. We normally have the knee flexed about 60° except during the last few weeks when we are remobilizing it with a hinged cast. As I mentioned, the hinged cast allows motion from $30^\circ - 60^\circ$. That is 30° of flexion to 60° of flexion. So we do keep the knee quite acutely flexed, even during the period of mobilisation.

O'DONOGHUE: I don't know just which part of Dr. MOSCHI'S presentation I should discuss. It is very interesting, but some of it is impracticable. I categorically cannot agree with some of the statements he made. I do not necessarily think 60° is the most relaxed position. I actually think it is about 30°. Most people say it is from $30^\circ - 60^\circ$. I prefer to use 30°, although many times it is 45°. Contrary to Dr. HUGHSTON'S experience, I have considerable difficulty in regaining extension if I hold the knee in 60° of flexion over a long period of time. Maybe there are more limber knees in Georgia than in Oklahoma. I am not sure about that.

Dr. MOSCHI also made a pretty categorical statement about where the injuries are. From my experience, the majority of injuries to the long fibers of the medial collateral ligament are below the knee, quite frequently under the pes, so that the tear is quite distal. Even with the deep capsular fibers, I think they are just as frequently torn below the meniscus as they are above. As a matter of fact, they are often torn both above and below. Of course, what we try to do is get the advancement far enough distally so that the level of the capsular ligament repair is actually on the tibia, hopefully getting a good fixation. Obviously, I do not think this superior advancement is as good as the inferior one that I have been doing, and I have been doing it for a long time. I believe MAUCK was the first one to describe advancing the medial collateral attachment with the block of bone. This is a great oversimplification of medial side instability. I think you need a more comprehensive reinforcement with all available material.

Another thing that you should bear in mind about the meniscus is that here, you are not dealing with a normal knee, as Dr. JAMES pointed out a few minutes ago. These knees are abnormal. I would say that in over half of my reconstruction cases the meniscus has already been removed before I see the patient. In the other 50%, I suppose 70% of the times the meniscus is abnormal. The only time the meniscus is not torn in when the tear is above the knee. In my experience the acute tear isolated above the knee is an infrequent injury. If the acute tear is above the joint, then it may require a simple repair with probably a better result than those that are more seriously damaged. I think the biomechanics is interesting, but I would sooner deal with the practicabilities and make a real effort to restore the ligament structures as nearly to normal as possible.

I would like to know how one knows when he has accurately restored the instant center and whether or not studies have been carried out following reconstruction in order to confirm the practicability of this theory.

I appreciate the discussion. We are here for an exchange of ideas so that each of us may profit by the others experiences and convictions.

MOSCHI: We have been working with the instant centers of rotation for other reasons besides ligamentous ones. However, we have been studying some instant centers of rotation in ligamentous injuries before surgery. In all cases the instant center of rotation was not normal, and that in my opinion is obvious. I do not have a sufficient follow-up of my patients to support that the function of the knee after surgery is normal. If I perform a reconstruction of the knee and try to obtain a normal instant center of rotation on that knee, I must take the opposite one as comparison. After a meniscectomy, for instance, I will have a fairly normal instant center of rotation, although it is very difficult to determine if it is normal or not. I sometimes have to perform a surgical reconstruction and must also take out a torn meniscus; sometimes they are not so badly instead torn that we must take them out extramurally but only have to take out the rim by an intramural meniscectomy, leaving some dynamic supports inside the knee joint just like in a normal meniscectomy. In that case I hope to have a normal instant center of rotation after surgery or at least more normal than before surgery. The most important part of the instant centers of rotation is from 60° on, because it is at that moment that the instant center of rotation comes close to the evolute. The center of rotation never arrives at the evolutes in a normal knee. I do not suppose that it will occur after reconstruction, but the closer it is to the evolute, the better the biomechanic knee function is.

JAMES: I think the important thing to remember with all these reconstructive procedures is the principle behind them. If you analyse them all, you will discover that the principles are very similar. Dr. O' DONOGHUE'S technique accomplishes what I accomplish with mine and what the Slocum technique also accomplishs. They are only simple modifications developed by different individuals who have found that their particular technique works in their own hands. I think that the technique which you selected may be modelled after one of these, or perhaps has been modified by you in a way that you find works for you. I think the important thing is to remember not so much the specific technique that we presented, but instead the principles behind the repair, i.e., taking up the medial side of the knee and then reinforcing it internally. I do not think that the type you used is necessarily dictated by whether or not the lesion basically was above or below the meniscus. It is the amount and type of instability which you can demonstrate during the preoperative examination that will dictate the application of the principles.

TREUMANN: Dr. JAMES, you were using prosthetic ligaments in medial repair. You employed prosthetic ligaments as SLOCUM did, doing the repair as you just described. Have you quit using it and are now using the Eriksson method instead?

JAMES: I have not been using the prosthetic ligament anteriorly; Dr. SLOCUM is now also using Eriksson for the anterior cruciate ligament in lieu of the prosthetic ligament. We found that using the prosthetic cruciate ligament anteriorly in replacement of the anterior cruciate ligament was not nearly as successful as using it in replacement of a posterior cruciate ligament. Right now we are looking for alternate means of substituting for the anterior cruciate ligament, but the important thing to remember is that any time you do reconstruction on the anterior cruciate ligament, whether it was a prosthetic ligament or of some other tissue, you must also do the additional repairs necessary around the periphery of the knee.

RITTMANN: You have recommended removing menisci for chronic instability Can you tell us whether you are as "aggressive" against the meniscus or not in cases where you are initially operating for primary repair?

JAMES: In the primary repair, I make every effort to preserve the medial meniscus. The reason that we recommend removing it with the reconstruction procedure is that we feel we are going to disrupt the mechanics of the meniscus to the extent that it will eventually develop problems and have to be removed secondarily. In the initial operation, I would if possible preserve it.

10. Anterior Subluxation of the Lateral Tibial Plateau

J.C.Kennedy

In our classification, anterolateral rotatory instability in the knee
may occur either in flexion or as the knee approaches extension. The
former condition, anterolateral rotatory instability in flexion, cor-
responds with its opposite number, the anteromedial rotatory instability that JAMES and SLOCUM have described so well. We do not think
that anterolateral rotatory instability in flexion is an important
instability. However, anterolateral rotatory instability as the knee
approaches extension has been popularized in North America by McINTOSH
with his description of the pivot shift test, by HUGHSTON with his
so-called jerk test, and finally by ELLISON who devised his rather
simple, ingenious operation of the fascia rerouting. I personally
would like to pay tribute to Dr. McINTOSH of Toronto for his astute
and original observation pertaining to the clinical entity of anterolateral rotatory instability as the knee approaches extension.
However, in the United States there has certainly been a great deal
of confusion as to the interpretation of the many features of anterior
subluxation of the lateral tibial plateau. These include problems
such as: What are the basic structural defects to produce this symptom?
What are the specific clinical tests? When are they positive? And
finally, what technique should you select to correct this disabling
entity?

I shall describe briefly the three tests for the clinical phenomenon.
The McIntosh test starts with the leg in extension, with a valgus
force being applied. In this position the tibia plateau has subluxed;
the subluxation reduces as the knee goes to 40^0 of flexion. Reduction
takes place as the knee flexes and dislocation, as the knee extends.
The second test is a so-called Losee test. We start this with the
knee in flexion and gradually produce some subluxation as the knee
approaches extension. The thumb is behind the fibula; the left fore-
fingers are secured around the patella to stop rotation; and the ankle
is cradled in the right arm. The subluxation occurs just as the knee
approaches extension. The third and final test, the Slocum maneuver
is a nice, subtle test for the apprehensive patient. Have the patient
lie on his sound side, up one hip, with the knee flexed. Gently apply
valgus force on the knee so that you can see the reduction in flexion
subluxation in extension, and anterior subluxation of the lateral
tibial plateau as the knee approaches extension.

I think that if one or all of these clinical tests is positive and
the patient without prompting recognizes this phenomena as his symp-
tomatology and his clinical problem, then the surgical indications
are present. If such a parallelism is not present, then the surgical
treatment is doomed to failure. All we are saying really is that when
you have carried out these tests, the patient has to say, "That's it!
That's what I feel; that's the way my knee gives way." If he doesn't
do this, I think you may often produce this test when it has no major
clinical significance. You must have a parallelism between the
patient's complaints and your clinical test.

Surgical Technique

I shall now discuss the operative technique which we employed to correct this disability on patients whom we operated during the period
between December 1974 and July 1976. I am not including recently
operated patients in my discussion so that I can relate follow-up
results to you. I am also not including another series of patients
operated during this same period for which we changed our technique
slightly.

We used this technique on 52 patients during the above-mentioned
period, 30 of whom we considered to have an isolated anterolateral
rotatory instability in extension. The remaining 22 patients had a
combination of simple anterolateral and anteromedial rotatory instability, and a pes anserinus transfer was necessary. Of these, 14 were
actually discarded either because of the employment of back-up procedures for major lateral knee joint reconstruction or because of an
overall operative procedure, such as the introduction of a synthetic
ligament.

The Ellison procedure appealed to us because we considered it a
simple, ingenious operation with dynamic potential. In many ways the
procedure mimics the original technique of McINTOSH in Toronto, but
it is in a reverse manner. The incision begins at the Gerdy's tubercle
and extends for a considerable distance up the lateral aspect of the
tigh, approximately 16 mm. Gerdy's tubercle is identified and removed,
including the insertion of the illiotibial tract. Care must be taken
at this stage not to enter the joint through the lateral tibial
plateau, i.e., you should not get your osteotomy cut too deep nor
fragment the piece of bone when performing the osteotomy of the tubercle. It is important, to broaden and widen your proximal portion
of the illiotibial band up to 4-5 cm width at its proximal attachment.
By doing so, it is hoped to preserve the blood supply of the illiotibial band and also to maintain the possibility of a dynamic function.

The portion of the illiotibial band at the joint line is reasonably
strong, being almost as strong as the original anterocruciate ligament. Frankly, during our instron laboratory testing, which we did
at a rate of physiological loading, we anticipated that the illiotibial tract would be much stronger than the anterior cruciate ligament. However, it is actually a little bit weaker than the anterior
cruciate ligament. A routine arthrotomy is always carried out through
the area from which the illiotibial tract has been delivered. One is
struck by the degree of thinness of the capsule in this area.

A quick evaluation is then carried out for structural deficit in the
anterior cruciate ligament, in the lateral meniscus, and for associated
condylar chondromalacia. We estimated that 95% of our patients had a
damaged anterior cruciate ligament, and frankly I think we could put
that up to 100% without being dogmatic. We found it necessary to remove the lateral meniscus because of obvious major tears in 44% of
the patients. Finally, 40% of our patients had visible and obvious
condylar chondromalacia of the lateral femoral condyle.

A most important step at this time is to insure the clearance of a
passage way just beneath the distal portion of the ligament. We feel
it is important not to free too much the fibular collateral ligament
and only the distal portion. If you dissect beneath the fascia at
this region (which is an easier method and frees the collateral liga-

ment), you end up with too generous a passage way for your rerouted
fascia, and you interfere with the posterior angulation of your transfer. So for this reason we only free the distal portion of the fibular
collateral ligament.

It is now important to undercut widely the anterior and posterior
margins of the remaining host fascia in preparation for adequate and
thorough closure of this region. Gerdy's tubercle with its attached
fascia is now rerouted beneath the fibular collateral ligament near
its fibular insertion; it is advanced and reattached distally. The
use of AO-compression screw nails with adequate reeinforcing sutures
has provided excellent fixation in our hands. Other people like to
use a staple. I have used a screw nail with reinforcing sutures and
for quite some time have had no cause to regret it.

Closure of this defect now becomes a major step; this is easily
achieved proximally where the nature of the tissue lends itself to
closure. As you approach the joint line it is often very difficult
to obtain adequate closure, and we often have to accomplish this by
slowly extending the knee as we tie the sutures. This step is of extreme importance since several authorities, including HUGHSTON,
ANDREWS, and others, consider a lateral capsular defect one of the
other contributing structural causes for anterolateral rotatory instability. In follow-up of the Ellison procedure we have noted that
several patients demonstrated one-plane lateral instability, which
was certainly due to inadequate closure of the fascia at the joint
line. In cases where anteromedial rotatory instability accompanies
anterior subluxation of the lateral tibial plateau, a pes anserinus
transfer is carried out and totally completed before the lateral side
is completed. Early in our series immobilization was carried out in
a neutral position following this dual procedure; however, we now
feel that we do not jeapordize the pes by immobilizing the combined
procedure in some 60^0 of flexion with external rotation and valgus.

Common Surgical Errors
=======================

Here are a few of the common technical errors. As I mentioned, in
removing Gerdy's tubercle one must be very cautious in not entering
the joint. Additional care must be taken to avoid fragmentation of
the small fragment of bone which must be passed beneath the fibular
collateral ligament and later fixed to the host tissue. We also feel
that the direction of the rerouted illiotibial band is most important.
On several occasions it has been necessary to reimplant the transfer
because of lack of proper angulation. As I pointed out, if the passage
way beneath the fibular collateral ligament has been created in too
generous a fashion, the posterior angulation of the transfer will be
lost; in such a case we consider the operation futile. The removal
of the fascia should be centered on the thickest portion of the illiotibial tract, leaving sufficant remaining posterior margin for an
adequate closure. The importance of securing adequate width cannot be
overemphasized. We feel it is rather nice to make your posterior cut
first. If you make the anterior cut first, the fascia will drop down;
for this reason we like to make a posterior cut in a fascia initially
and then to move up and cut the anterior fascia. At the proximal
level, the width of the transfer should be 4.5 cm. Once again, we
must stress the danger of producing residual one-plane lateral instability if there is not an adequate lateral compartment closure. We
must once again emphasize how very important this is, although this

portion of the operation takes perhaps just as long as the entire remainder of the procedure.

I mentioned that in postoperative care the position of the knee is 60-70° of flexion with abduction and external rotation. The cast is applied from toes to groin and must be rigidly inspected during the first 48 hours. The danger of a tight fascial closure must be emphasized, since it may cause a compartment syndrome. We all know about the vulnerability of the common peroneal nerve in this region.

Results of Surgical Treatment

As we mentioned, our follow-up was carried out on some 52 patients who underwent this procedure between December 1974 and July 1976. We would like to caution you on any optimistic conclusions for this or any other series dealing with reconstructive knee surgery. I mentioned that an accurate assessment of results cannot be made until at least 10 years following corrective procedures about the knee joint. I think we should all remember our previous discussion of operative techniques in which it was clearly demonstrated in a series of 50 so-called isolated tears of the anterior cruciate ligament. To recapitulate, 80% of these were good or excellent at the 44 months period, whether or not surgically treated. This figure at 85 months had deteriorated to a failure rate of 35%, again with no statistical relationship to the type of surgical treatment. In an effort towards simplicity, we classified surgical results in one evaluation according to the patients' opinions. We asked whether they thought the operation was poor, fair, good, or excellent. We defined poor as being worse than before surgery; fair, only moderately improved; good, active in sport with caution; and excellent had unrestricted activity. Only 58% of our patients had a good or excellent result. Our review indicated that better selectivity and an improved surgical technique would unquestionably improve the results. We then reviewed our trends towards failure. A careful analysis of the patients revealed that a patient with a major positive anterior drawer sign (which we classify as being over 10 mm in association with clinical evidence of anterior subluxation of the lateral tibia plateau) will not be helped by the Ellison procedure alone. I think, this is important. Do not do this operation in an effort to cure the patient if he has a straight one-plane anterior drawer sign over 1 cm. Unfortunately, the prognosis for patients over 40 years of age was also not good, particularly if there was a delay between the initial injury and the time of our operation. If associated complicated instabilities are to be corrected, then the Ellison procedure should just be done as a part of a two-stage procedure. Do not do the Ellison and try to combine it with a major reconstruction on the inner side of the knee.

Technical errors as outlined previously reduce the success rate, as expected in the evolution of any new surgical technique. The two major causes and technical errors were: (1) difficulty in securing proper posterior angulation of the illiotibial tract, resulting in a defective dynamic force exerted against the anterior tibial subluxation, and (2) inability to close properly the host defect in the illiotibial tract.

Trends not affecting the failure were twofold. Firstly, the success
rate was not influenced by how grossly positive the so-called pivot
shift or anterior subluxation clinical test was. In other words, you
could have a major positive jerk test, pivot shift test, or anterior
subluxation test, and the surgical results were still not effected.
They were just as good, providing there was no major anterior drawer
sign. Secondly, an anterior subluxation operation combined with the
surgical treatment of an anteriormedial rotatory instability by way
of a pes anserinus transfer predictably could be handled successfully
with this combined procedure. In other words, combining the Ellison
procedure with a pes anserinus transfer did not cause any increase in
our failure rate.

Of 30 patients undergoing an Ellison procedure alone for anterior subluxation of the lateral tibial plateau 58% were good or excellent.
Of 22 patients undergoing an Ellison procedure and a pes anserinus
for combined anteromedial and anterolateral rotatory instability, the
success rate was approximately the same. Therefore, we concluded that
the Ellison procedure is a technically attractive transfer in the control of anterior subluxation of the lateral tibial plateau. The success rate for good or excellent reflects the need for extreme selectivity in the employment of the procedure. Eliminating technical
errors and improper indications in the group of 52 patients just discussed improved greatly the results in an ensuing group of 50 patients
that we have just recently completed. In patients with a positive or
grossly positive anterior drawer sign, the high failure rate suggests
that the Ellison procedure should not be used alone. To this end,
further reconstructive techniques have been conceived and introduced.
Such patients are now undergoing similar reviews.

11. Posterolateral Instability

A. Trillat

We are only dealing with purely ligamentous instabilities with no damage to cartilage and bones in the original trauma. Posterolateral instabilities have more devastating functional consequences than other types of instabilities. The stability of the knee is always disturbed, sometimes to such an extent that the patient can only walk with the aid of one or two canes.

There can be two occasions for these instabilities:

(1) Automobile dashboard injuries with the knee in 90° flexion, with posterior luxation on the tibial plateau. This trauma is often associated with multiple other lesions, which explains that the knee lesion quite often has not been formerly diagnosed. Thus, very late treatment is started only after the patient discovers that he has chronic instability of the knee.

(2) Sport accidents often due to collison with the opponent. The knee is deformed by adduction and exaggerated rotation. Often there is a complex lesion from the very beginning. The lateral pentad shows rupture or disattachment of the two cruciate ligaments, of the posterolateral capsule, of the lateral meniscus and of the lateral ligament. These are lesions with which an elongation of the lateral popliteal sciatic nerve and of the iliotibial tract, etc. can be associated.

Of course these lesions are in most cases treated immediately; therefore, most of the patients who come because of posterolateral instability have already been operated on. As a result the problem of an anterior incision and repairs done earlier can be associated with the problem of treating the instability.

Clinical Aspects and Examination Methods

The clinical picture is in general obvious: a functional instability is usually the patient's greatest handicap. One can almost say that if a patient complains of great instability, a posterolateral instability can be diagnosed. The pain is not constant and often reveals a meniscal lesion, as in cases of temporary hydrops.

A physical examination is essential for establishing local and general findings and must be methodical and determinative for each symptom.

Lateral instability is considered as
-in extension with
    zero
    +
    ++ and more

-in slight flexion of some 15° with the foot
    in neutral position
    in internal rotation
    in external rotation,
    (estimate the degree +, ++ or more)

-in certain cases one can see these displacements on X-rays taken in extreme varus and valgus positions.

The posterior drawer sign is normally detected when the knee is in a 90° flexion position or a little less. It is classified by +, ++, or more pluses and is tested in the three rotation positions (internal, neutral and external). It must also be tested at very slight flexion of approximately 15°. The frequency and exactness of its detection has grown considerably. Confusion can arise if one does not become aware of the fact that the knee being tested is chronicly posteriorly displaced. When one tries to find the anterior drawer sign, the tibia comes forward; however, this is just a correction.

Complementary examinations
-morphotype of the knee
    varus or valgus
    recurvation, very important to detect and to codify the height of
    the patella

-above
    muscular atrophy
    condition of the hip and the vertebral column

-below
    skin troubles, circulatory
    complete neurological and muscular examination

X-rays are an important aid in diagnosis. Besides X-rays of the positions indicated above, one should concentrate on the valgus and varus following positions. An X-ray in profile shows the status of the eminentia intercondylaris and the osseous zone situated behind it, as well as any small ossifications towards the middle of the knee or above the posterior cruciate ligament. A frontal view shows the status of the eminentia intercondylaris and the articular surfaces.

Xerography is costly, but we consider it a useful diagnostic aid. On the other hand we feel that arthrography is only of interest for purposes of documentation.

Surgical Treatment
==================

It is difficult to treat this instability surgically! On the medial side of the knee, multiple ligamentous and tendinous formations supply all the material necessary for reconstruction. On the lateral side the tendinous formations are either too weak e.g. the biceps muscle or too important to be deprived of their function (e.g. tensor muscle of fascia lata).

Applying a similar technique from the lateral side to that of O'DONOGHUE from the medial side, and at the same time adapting other ideas from the literature - it is difficult to determine who was the first to come up with a useful idea - the treatment of these lateral instabilities is carried out in our clinic as follows:

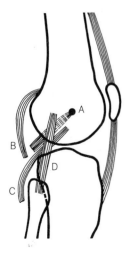

Fig. 1. (A) Origin of posterior cruciate ligament. This has been severed at its lower end (see B). (B) Inferior part of the posterior medial ligament rejoined by the posterial cruciate ligament, both of which are severed from the tibia. (C) Course of the popliteal muscle, the upper end of which will be fixed in the area of the lateral ligament. This muscle and its tendon are relaxed. (D) The fibular collateral ligament, relaxed

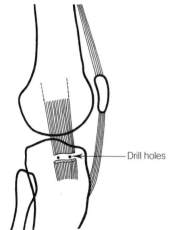

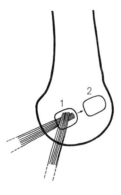

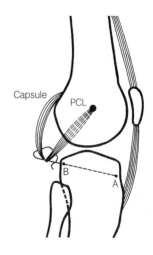

Fig. 2   Fig. 3   Fig. 4

Fig. 2. Iliotibial tract severed in the middle and horizontally at its tibial insertion. After the anterior horn of the lateral meniscus is severed, the lateral surfaces of the lateral tibial plateau and the femoral condyle can be exposed. This allows removal of the lateral meniscus as well as a view of the intercondylar incisure and the end of the tendon of the popliteal muscle. This cut also makes it easy to reconstruct the iliotibial tract with simple sutures

Fig. 3. Repositioning of the button of bone which includes the popliteal muscle and lateral ligament. After lifting of the synovial flap covering the insertion of the popliteal muscle and lateral ligament, (1) the button of bone with these two insertions is cut out. (2) Another block of the same size is cut out above and anterior to first button, which is then transposed to the prepared surface 2 and fixed by means of a clamp. The whole area is then covered again with the synovial flap

Fig. 4. After cutting out the button of bone (see Fig. 3), but before reconstructing the lateral side, the popliteal zone on the posterior surface of the tibia is prepared. Sutures are passed through the junction of the posterior capsule and the posterior cruciate ligament. These sutures are then threaded through the 2 or 3 drill holes from B to A; finally, they are likewise used to close up the severed iliotibial tract (see Fig. 2)

(1) A parapatellar lateral cutanous incision is made, passing just above the patella's superior border, descending along the patella tendon, and turning slightly posteriorly.

(2) The fascia lata is lifted, transversally cut in the middle of its insertion, and separated above and below from the retinacula so that some contact with the bone is maintained and good fixation is ensured.

(3) The soft tissue flap, including the fascia, synovium and the lateral meniscus up to the superior point of the fibula are turned back.

(4) A general lateral meniscectomy is undertaken. The lateral meniscus is often damaged, often intact. In either case it must be removed as it does not recover its physiology.

(5) Exposure of the tendon of the popliteal muscle.

(6) Exposure of the tendon of the lateral collateral ligament.

(7) Lifting of the synovial flap which covers it.

(8) A button of bone is cut out that includes the insertion of the popliteal muscle and the fibular collateral ligament.

(9) Exposure of the posterior face of the tibial plateau in the popliteal zone to allow passage of the posterior sutures, 2 to 4 small tunnels are drilled.

(10) The distal and posterior part of the posterior cruciate ligament is exposed, and the fixation sutures are passed through the drill holes.

(11) Transtibial tunnels are drilled according to O'DONOGHUE'S method. The tibia is penetrated at the level of the first incision of the fascia lata.

(12) The sutures are passed from the posterior zone through the tunnels.

(13) Exposure above and in front of the bony square detached from the external condyle, to allow the transposition in front of and above the detached square.

(14) The button of bone is fixed by means of a staple (including the insertion of the popliteal muscle and the fibular collateral ligament).

(15) Closure is achieved by utilizing transosseous sutures to reconstruct the initial insertion of the fascia lata.

(16) Suction drainage is applied to the wound, and a plaster cast is made.

The postoperative procedures are simple:

A large plaster cast from toe to groin is used for 10-15 days, after which time a double shell knee plaster cast is applied which allows locomotion with full load after 15 days. The knee cast is removed after 45 days. Progressive and, above all, active rehabilition is necessary over a period of time.

Results

The possibility of success of this operation is directly related to the position of the initial lesions. Failure is certain if the upper part of the posterior cruciate ligament is destroyed or ruptured. The large original incision allows for easy recognition of gross lesions to the posterior cruciate ligament. Should such lesions in its upper part be discovered upon first inspection, a different solution must be found for this knee.

Badly healed lesions of the fibular collateral ligament below do not allow the utilization of the described method, but in certain cases it is possible to regain hold of the popliteal muscle above and to retain the fibular collateral ligament below. However, this last point is difficult to carry out, and the results are poor.

Severe lesions of the popliteal muscle are the cause of all failures. In this case the proposed method is no longer applicable. We have tried passive transplantation according to the Lindemann procedure, but I remain convinced that the moment the popliteal ligament is destroyed, every result - regardless of which method is applied - is inevitably going to be poor.

For cases, however, in which the lower part of the posterior cruciate ligament has been ruptured and the upper part of the fibular collateral ligament and in which the popliteal muscle is not traumatized, the proposed method has proven so successful that it allows young athletes to return to sports in 10 out of 11 cases.

Discussion

JAKOB: I would like to ask you three questions: (1) What is necessary if there is no posterior cruciate ligament? (2) Why do you mobilize a knee already one week after the operation? There are cases where a new instability occurs because of too early mobilization. (3) With how many kilos do you load the knee cast after two weeks?

TRILLAT: (1) The suppression or the disappearance of the posterior cruciate ligament is much more seldom than the disappearance of the anterior cruciate ligament. Therefore this problem does not occur so often.

(2) Up to now we do not know which is the best way of reconstructing the posterior cruciate ligament. Therefore we tried to use artificial ligaments which from a surgical point of view are extremely easy to implant and which restore stability to the knee within six months. Unfortunately, after 4 or 5 years of use there were many problems which confronted us: firstly, a chronic joint hydrops; secondly, a rupture of the artificial ligament; and thirdly, in 3 out of 50 cases, a necrosis of the cartilage of the internal femoral condyle due to excessive pressure and tension of this artificial posterior cruciate ligament. These problems must be investigated in research centers, and we presently cannot say where our preferences will lie. I am convinced that within the next few weeks the good results that we obtained in some 60% of the cases will lead us to new attempts. If you apply the described tests there will be practically no abnormal mobility in the first 6 weeks after operation. Everything else is depending on follow-up studies; therefore, I do not think that early mobilisation provokes a rapid instability of the knee. If this is the case, the method has to be abandoned.

(3) Eight days after the operations one sees the patients walking without assistance and without a cane. The knee is stiff because of a
plaster cast. I personally attach great importance to these operative
consequences not only because of the fact that the patient can flex
the knee soon, but because this is a hard test for the surgical method
one has applied, and also because such surgery does not lead to good
anatomical results. If there is instability the moment the plaster is
removed and the patient uses the knee, it is perhaps due to too early
mobilisation. However, if this instability does not occur and the patient did walk at an early stage, this speaks in favor of the method.

MÜLLER: Since you are now performing this new operation, have you completely abandoned the former method where the fibular head was transposed to a position in front of the tibia?

TRILLAT: This operative procedure was used for anterolateral instabilities about 10 years ago. Since then we have more classifications of
knee instabilites, and knee examinations have become much more detailed.
If this intervention is to be used, it can only be applied in cases of
anterolateral instability without any posterolateral instability.

RITTMANN: Dr. KENNEDY, what is your treatment for posterolateral instability?

KENNEDY: We treat posterolateral instability very poorly. In North
America Professor TRILLAT had only 11 cases on which he was reporting
with a 2-year follow-up. It is not a common instability in North America
Not many of us have advanced the origin of the femoral attachment of
the popliteal muscle. Most of our reconstructions have been on the arcuate ligament complex. I must admit that our results do not compare
when I hear Professor TRILLAT say that he can get 10 of 11 patients
back to athletics and tennis with his technique. I think we should pay
attention to it. Most of our attacks have been attempting to pull the
posterolateral corner of the tibia forward by some sort of tightening
of the arcuate ligament complex rather than a detailed attack on the
origin of the popliteal muscle or insertion whichever you prefer.

O'DONOGHUE: I have done this advancement as part of an overall Gerdy
lateral side reconstruction, via taking off the illiotibial band and
Gerdy's tubercle; this was possible because I have been taking it off
as a strip of fascia, pulling it downwards, and then pulling it up
again later. Our method is to strip off the whole femoral condyle on
the lateral side, very much as we strip off the medial tibia. That includes the popliteus and the fibular collateral ligament and also the
posterior capsule. As a result you can pull the whole thing up, put
the drill holes on the femur, and finally fasten the whole flap proximally as far as it will go. The results on the lateral side are not
as good in my hands as those of the medial side, with which I am very
satisfied. The lateral side can perhaps be improved by Professor TRIL-
LAT'S technique.

JAKOB: Is this operation also favorable in a recurved idiopathic, non-
tramatic knee?

TRILLAT: In a recurvation due to congenital instability or instability
of the poliomyelitic type, the problem is a completely different one.

SCHULITZ: How do you proceed in a combined lateral and medial complex
instability?

TRILLAT: Where there is a combined medial and lateral instability, we
are dealing with completely different types of knees. There are various

possibilities. I personally think that it is better to operate the most injured side first and then the less injured side. If you want to dismantle completely the superior extremity of the tibia posteriorly and laterally, you run the risk of a necrosis of the tibia. We had two cases of necrosis of the tibia when we started the operation with the internal side and combined it with the external side, as Dr. O'DONOGHUE does. Therefore we are very cautious about bilateral operations. If, however, a Slocum transplantation is to be performed, this does not imply great difficulties. However, if a severe internal instability exists, I am not sure whether the Slocum method is sufficient. Dr. KENNEDY'S statistics on anterolateral instabilities show that in the two groups where (a) only the lateral side is operated on (b) the lateral side plus the Slocum operation are carried out, there are practically no differences of the late results.

JAKOB: I still have one more comment to the method of Dr. KENNEDY, who kindly mentioned the work of MCINTOSH. In contrast to the Ellison modification, the original method of MCINTOSH'S lateral substitution repair is a purely static one, using a strip of the fascia lata, leading it under the upper part of the fibular collateral ligament, and then threading it through an osteoperiostal tunnel to the intermuscular septum. In cases where we were not satisfied with the degree of fixation of the ligament, we have used slight modifications by tightening it with an AO screw. Some people say that this repair is really purely static and fascial and may become loose in time. The Ellison procedure has the advantage that it is a dynamic repair, but as I heard from Dr. JAMES, some people are not always happy because it, too, may become loose. Now to combine the two effects of these two procedures, we have started using a combination of them using anteriorly the original McIntosh method and for the posterior part, of the iliotibial tract, taking off a piece of Gerdy's tubercle, very much in the way Dr. KENNEDY has shown. If MCINTOSH has about 70% good results with his method and Dr. KENNEDY about 60% with his, I think we may achieve up to 130% good results with our method.

12. Isolated Tear of the Anterior Cruciate Ligament

M. E. Blazina

The topic to be discussed has already been mentioned several times at this meeting, i.e., the so-called "isolated tear of the anterior cruciate ligament". This entity was vigorously described by Mr. MURDOCH of Dundee, Scotland, in about 1956. He was a colleague of Professor SMILLIE, who himself felt that this lesion was not really isolated but occurred because of impingement phenomena most probably related to meniscal pathology. About 1970 in the United States, two groups, perhaps working synchronously, began to emphasize the lesion of the isolated tear of the anterior cruciate ligament. One group was located at West Point, New York, representing the U.S. Military Academy. The other group was located in Atlanta, Georgia, headed by Dr. FRED ALLMAN. They both initially described a surprisingly high incidence of these lesions, espesially Dr. ALLMAN. Later on, after some of the early investigators had left West Point, having been transferred elsewhere as career officers, the incidence appeared to decline.

Criteria for Possible Diagnosis

In order to evaluate properly this entity, it is important that we delineate the lesion exactly as described by its principal investigators so that you may compare your impression with that as outlined at West Point. According to West Point doctors, an isolated tear of the anterior cruciate ligament is a diagnosis which is:

Primarily	related to acute knee injuries,
Possibly	related to a subacute knee problem, and
Rarely	related to chronic knee derangement.

In order to fulfill all the criteria of an "isolated tear of the anterior cruciate ligament" as described by the West Point group, six components must be present:

1. A "pop" at the time of injury, i.e., the patient feels a very definite snap in the knee.
2. This discrete injury must be a disabling phenomenon, i.e., the patient is absolutely unable to continue his activity.
3. Gross swelling via hemarthrosis occurs within 12 hours, a point forcefully stressed by COLONEL FEAGIN, one of the principal investigators.
4. The injury occurs without contact, either with an object or another player. Instead, the injury occurs in a deceleration phase, usually while trying to change direction. The player is running, suddenly decides to slow down and turn, becomes confused, and injures his knee
5. No other clinical diagnosis is apparent after a thorough search of both compartments of the knee through a rather small anteromedial incision.
6. At the time of their original presentation, the investigators stated that there was no detectable instability in the knee. Recent opinions

have been that one can detect slight anteroposterior play, especially with a stress machine such as that described by Dr. KENNEDY.

Using the above criteria, the investigators noted a rather high incidence of this lesion. Dr. ALLMAN, for instance, at one time stated
that one-third of all the ligamentous injuries of the knee that he
encountered in a single year were isolated tears of the anterior cruciate ligament. (This impression seemed to be incompatible with the
observations of most other orthopedists in the United States who were
seeing similar types of injuries.) Also, the West Point group and Dr.
ALLMAN stated that in their early postoperative evaluations that they
were having excellent results with direct repair of the torn anterior
cruciate ligament. Many of these patients went back to American football, and many others were able to stay in the Army, being apparently
capable of fulfilling the rigid physical requirements of the U.S. Army.

Certain subsequent events occurred. As stated above, many of the initial
investigators left West Point. Their successors did not find an incidence of this lesion anywhere near that of the original group. The
introduction of arthrography and arthroscopy as part of the workup obviated some of the limitations of the small anteromedial arthrotomy
incision, and other lesions besides the torn anterior cruciate ligament were noted. For instance, Dr. KENNEDY in discussing one of the
original papers, mentioned associated tears of the lateral meniscus.
Semantically, it would be difficult to accept a diagnosis of "isolated
tear of the anterior cruciate ligament plus a torn lateral meniscus".
Parenthetically, although unknown at the time, some of Dr. KENNEDY'S
cases may also have had anterolateral instability.

At the time of the introduction of the entity of the isolated tear of
the anterior cruciate ligament in 1970 or 1971, there existed in the
United States an almost nihilistic attitude toward the anterior cruciate
ligament. The feeling existed that the anterior cruciate ligament just
did not play an important role; therefore why all the hullabaloo about
a torn anterior cruciate ligament? No specific treatment was indicated
anyhow. At the present time in 1977, especially as discussed at this
meeting, the feeling exists that the anterior cruciate ligament is a
very important ligament, that it has significant functions, and that,
if possible, it should be repaired or reconstructed.

In a subsequent article with more prolonged follow-up, COLONEL FEAGIN
recently reported a different set of results than those initially reported. The article appeared in the American Journal of Sports Medicine,
a publication of the American Orthopedic Society for Sports Medicine,
an organization founded by Dr. O'DONOGHUE six years ago. In that article, COLONEL FEAGIN stated that the results were no longer so favorable. Instead of the initial 90%-95% excellent results, after 5 years
only about 30% had a satisfactory result. Over 70% had begun to note
the development of significant symptoms. According to his report, something dynamically was happening to these knees:

Progressive deterioration of knee function, probably because of secondary attritional stretching of juxta-articular supporting structures
(capsule and ligaments)

Ultimate tears of one or both menisci

Eventual articular cartilage damage

The incompetence of the anterior cruciate ligament may even be a cau-
sative factor in malfunctioning of extensor mechanism.

Our united experience appears to give a similar impression (Table 1).

Table 1. Surgery on anterior cruciate ligament

A. ACL repair (6 cases)
   Subsequent surgery (1 case)
      Medial meniscectomy
      Anteromedial and posteromedial capsular reefings

B. Excision of tag of ACL (16 cases)
   Subsequent surgery (4 cases)
      Medial meniscectomy
      Pes anserinus transfer
      ACL reconstruction (Jones)
      Anterolateral capsular reefing

      Medial meniscectomy
      Anteromedial and posteromedial capsular reefing
      Pes anserinus transfer
      Lateral meniscectomy
      Modified Ellison procedure

      Lateral meniscectomy
      Chondroplasties of lateral femoral condyle and intercondylar eminence

      Vastus medialis transposition
      Vastus lateral release
      Lateral meniscectomy

Possible Treatment

The question we have to ask ourselves, having reviewed the above information, is, "How aggressive should we be in approaching an early case of a torn anterior cruciate ligament?" Despite the possibility that perhaps only 30% of the cases have a satisfactory result with direct repair, knowing the possible consequences after a development of chronic anterior instability, we must ask ourselves whether it is still not worthwhile to repair torn anterior cruciate ligaments? Also, perhaps we should reinforce with fascia lata or patellar tendon those tears most unfavorable for repair alone, such as midsubstance tears and avulsions of the anterior cruciate ligament near or at its femoral attachment. Of course, in deciding how aggressive we should be toward an early tear of the anterior cruciate ligament, we should be aware of how much stress the patient may potentially place on that knee in the future. Certainly, a young athlete most probably will try to remain active. If he does, we may expect that the second line of defense, i.e., the juxta-articular supporting structures, will have to assume the load. Secondary attrition and stretching of these structures may occur, along with progressive deterioration of knee function including articular cartilage damage and patellar dysfunction. Wouldn't it be better to obviate this phenomenon if at all possible?

The isolated tear of the anterior cruciate ligament is an intriguing lesion with many important considerations. At the present time we certainly do not have all the answers. However, it is hoped that by the above discussion we will agree not to disregard it or to consider it lightly.

13. Prosthetic Ligaments – Indications

M. E. Blazina

It is important to adopt a definite philosophical attitude towards ligamentous reconstruction of the knee. In initiating the concept of a synthetic ligament, one's mentality must also be synchronized with the accompanying concept of "failure." If all repairs of acute ligamentous tears turned out well, one would not encounter failure and, therefore, one would not need to consider developing a prosthetic ligament. Likewise, if all reconstructions of the ligamentous instabilities of the knee utilizing autogenous structures turned out well, one would not encounter failure and, therefore, one would not need to consider developing a synthetic ligament.

Somewhere, sometime, we must talk about "failure." This has not been done in our country. There has been reported a series of acute posterior cruciate ligament repairs with 27 out of 29 excellent results without any discussion as to the need for future surgery. There is no place for a synthetic ligament in that kind of discussion. There has been reported a series of medial side reconstructions with 96% of the cases reported as having obtained full preinjury functional status with no apparent need for further surgery. There is no place in that particular context for a synthetic ligament.

On the other hand, rational evaluation of surgical experiences should reveal to us that failure does indeed exist, and in knee surgery as a totality it may approach somewhere around 20%-25%. If we do concide failure of some acute ligamentous repairs and of some chronic ligamentous reconstructions, then we must be prepared to concede failure of some of the synthetic ligaments. One will not be universally sucesful there either.

Following along this pattern of thought, at no time would the insertion of a prosthetic ligament be considered as a substitute procedure for autogenous reconstruction. At one time we were concerned about chronic posterior instability, but, as indicated by Dr. KENNEDY, that thinking has changed since the introduction of the prosthetic ligament, and we ourselves will elaborate on this entity further on. Another aspect for consideration when dealing with autogenous versus prosthetic ligament reconstruction is the concept that one should work doubly hard to improve autogenous ligament reconstruction, thus avoiding the necessity for using prosthetic ligaments. This very situation has occurred in the last five years. Our understanding of both anterior and posterior instability has been increased. Improved autogenous procedures, especially for anterolateral and posterolateral instability have been recently developed. There has been a renaissance of anterior cruciate ligament reconstruction utilizing the patellar tendon. Each step forward in this direction obviates the need for synthetic ligaments. Reluctance at this stage to utilize prosthetic ligaments also rests upon the fact that with insertion of a synthetic ligament, we would automatically relegate the patient to a discrete subfunctional level. Our problem is similar to that of the dentist. If he can save one's teeth, that is always more preferrable than installing a set of false dentures with their own masticatory limitations.

Insofar as anterior instability is concerned, current thinking would
appear to indicate that if anteromedial instability alone exists, then
we have the procedures available to handle this situation and should
do so. If anterolateral instability alone exists, then we have the
procedures available to handle this situation and should do so, if combined anteromedial and anterolateral instability exists, then we should
be prepared to operate on both sides of the knee at the same sitting.
Finally, as suggested by Dr. KENNEDY, if anteromedial and anterolateral
instability coexist with significant single-plane anterior instability,
we should be prepared to stabilize the knee medially, laterally, and
in the middle - all at one time. An approach such as this will increase our success rate and significantly lessen the need for prosthetic
ligaments.

Insofar as indications for the use of a prosthetic anterior cruciate
ligament are concerned, we would not consider using a prosthetic ligament for acute tears of the anterior cruciate ligament (Table 1). In

Table 1. Indications for prostetic anterior cruciate ligaments

---

1. Acute tears of ACL:<u>no</u>

2. Initial approach to chronic anterior instability:<u>no</u>

3. Secondary approach to chronic anterior instability:<u>not if alternative procedures
   available</u>

4. Tertiary approach to chronic anterior instability:<u>consider if</u>

   a) No other alternative procedures available

   b) Knee progressively deteriorating

   c) Other coexisting instability components can also be taken care of especially
      rotatory components; otherwise ligament will fail

---

fact, from the lessons learned in studying the so-called isolated anterior cruciate ligament tear," it would appear that we should seriously consider reinforcement via the use of a strip of the patellar
tendon or the iliotibial band at the time of anterior cruciate ligament
repair. Perhaps that way we can obtain a functional anterior cruciate
ligament and avoid the possible consequences of having a knee with a
nonfunctioning anterior cruciate ligament. That would represent an
ideal situation.

We have already described our initial approach to chronic anterior instability. If our initial approach fails, it does so most probably because we did not do enough, and the situation may still be salvageable
utilizing augmenting autogenous procedures.

If our secondary approach fails, we have then reached a predicament.
We usually have exhaused effective autogenous procedures; the knee
is progressively deteriorating insofar as the articular cartilage is
concerned; and the patient is usually young, functionally disabled,
and in considerable discomfort. We have reached a desperate situation
and are really seriously considering arthrodesis. The patient is reluctant to accept fusion and consequently may be ready to accept some
other alternative such as a prosthetic ligament. If the prosthetic
ligament could stabilize the knee, even if only for a limited period
of time, perhaps at the end of that time we will have sufficiently
advanced technologically to keep the knee moving in a satisfactory
manner. On the other hand, once a knee is fused, the quadriceps mechanism becomes nonfunctional. Reversing a fusion would represent a   ·
formidable procedure.

Table 2. Indications for posterior cruciate ligaments

1. Acute tears of PCL:<u>no</u>

2. Initial approach to chronic posterior instability:

   a) <u>Not if</u> one feels instability can be handled by doing juxta-articular procedures alone

   b) <u>Not if</u> one feels PCL reconstruction can be done using autogenous structures

   c) Consider <u>if</u> one feels that the instability cannot be handled by doing juxta-
   articular procedures alone <u>and if</u> one feels that autogenous reconstruction
   will be insufficient

3. Secondary approach to chronic posterior instability:

   a) <u>Consider</u> especially <u>if</u> have no other approach available and knee is de-
   toriating

   b) <u>Must</u> complement with juxta-articular procedures or else prosthetic ligament
   alone will be unsatisfactory and/or fail

The story of chronic posterior instability of the knee is a peculiar
one (Table 2). Certain changes in attitude toward posterior instability
are occurring at the present time, but if one reviews past attitudes,
one is impressed by the almost nihilistic attitude that was assumed
several years ago. The standard textbooks on knee surgery avoided any
discussion of autogenous procedures for chronic posterior instability.
There were spokesmen for the extremely conservative nonoperative approach, consisting essentially and quadriceps exercises. Others were
known to feel that the chronic posterior instability really did not
contribute to noticeable loss of knee function.

Significant chronic posterior instability of the knee is indeed disabling! One cannot start or stop suddenly. One has considerable difficulty walking downhill or down an incline. The natural history of
chronic posterior instability leads to progressive deterioration of
the menisci and the articular cartilages of the medial and lateral
compartments. The patellofemoral articulation is working at a mechanical
disadvantage due to the posterior sag of the tibia and will develop
chondromalacic changes sooner or later.

It has become apparent recently that there are several planes of posterior instability, just as described above as occurring in anterior
instability. Posteromedial instability does exist but does not represent the same degree of problem as its counterpart, posterolateral
instability. Anterior instabilites also may be present along with posterior instabilities.

What comes up for consideration is the possibility that in the past,
trying to stabilize posterior instability by routing a tendon such as
the semitendinosus through the middle of the knee represented an insufficient approach to the total problem of posterior instability. It
may very well be that by combining autogenous posterior cruciate ligament reconstruction with posterolateral and posteromedial stabilization (or whatever else is needed), will improve our results in these
cases. On the other hand, if despite this combined approach it becomes
quite apparent that the autogenous structures utilized as posterior
cruciate ligament substitutes are biomechanically insufficient to stabilize the knee, then we will seriously have to consider "backing-up"
the above-mentioned procedures with a synthetic ligament as suggested
by Dr. SLOCUM and Dr. KENNEDY (Table 2).

In a recent review of 25 cases of autogenous posterior cruciate ligament reconstruction done by us (Table 3), it was noted that 7 patients
required a secondary operation (Table 2). Some of these reconstructions

Table 3. Posterior cruciate ligament reconstructions

1. Methods of reconstruction

Semitendinosus	9
Posteromedial capsule	4
Semimembranosus	3
Medial meniscus	3
Lateral meniscus	3
Medial head of gastrocnemius	2
Vastus medialis obliquus	1
	25

2. Patients needing subsequent surgery
   7/25 (28%)

3. Subsequent procedures

Lateral meniscectomy	4
Medial meniscectomy	2
Partial synovectomy	2
Pes anserinus transfer	2
Posterolateral capsular reefing	1
Iliotibial band advancement	1
Forward transposition of lateral head of gastrocnemius	1
Biceps tendon transfer to lateral femoral epicondyle	1
Arthrodesis of knee	1
Miscellaneous	11
	26

were deficient because of significant residual posterolateral instability. We were most interested in hearing about Professor TRILLAT'S
operation for posterolateral instability, as it may represent a distinct advance in handling this particularly difficult problem.

We would also like to point out that until a synthetic ligament is
developed that will control rotation, there will always be a need for
stabilization both posteromedially and posterolaterally. In fact, by
stabilizing the knee in the neutral plane, we actually may be accent-
ing even further the rotatory instabilities.

In reviewing the subsequent procedures for the synthetic ligaments
utilized as a prosthetic anterior cruciate ligament, there are several
considerations to be noted (Table 4). First of all, some of the secondary procedures were not all related to instability itself, such as the
removal of methylmethacrylate or a loose body. On the other hand, there
were definite episodes of breakage of the prosthetic ligament. Some
of these cases could be attributed to the technique and site of insertion rather than a biomechanic deficiency of the ligament itself. Some
of these cases, especially those done early in the series, were definitely related to our insufficient understanding of anterolateral
instability. Lastly, it can be noted that some patients went on to
replacement surgery, i.e., articular cartilage was already present in
a far-advanced stage, and there was a need to cover the articular surfaces.

Table 4. Prosthetic anterior cruciate ligaments

1. Patients needing subsequent surgery
   $\frac{14}{45}$ (30%)

2. Subsequent procedures

Removal of prosthetic ACL	5
Ellison procedure	3
Release of intra-articular adhesions	3
Secondary lateral meniscectomy	2
Secondary prosthetic ACL	2
Biceps transfer to lateral femoral epicondyle	2
Chondroplasty of femoral groove	2
Chondroplasty of lateral femoral condyle	2
Lateral meniscectomy	2
Pes anserinus transfer	1
Removal of methylmethacrylate anterior compartment	1
Removal of methylmethacrylate suprapatellar pouch	1
Patellofemoral replacement	1
Lateral compartment replacement	1
Biceps forward	1
Secondary femoral nut - prosthetic ACL	1
Secondary Ellison procedure	1
Miscellaneous	9
	40

Table 5. Prosthetic posterior cruciate ligaments

1. Patients needing subsequent surgery
   $\frac{5}{14}$ (36%)

2. Subsequent procedures

Medial compartment replacement	2
Prosthetic medial collateral ligament	2
Removal of prosthetic PCL	2
Ellison procedure	1
Biceps transfer to lateral femoral epicondyle	1
Secondary prosthetic PCL	1
PFR	1
Tertiary prosthetic PCL	1
Reverse modified Ellison procedure	1
Arthrodesis of knee	1
PCL reconstruction (vastus medialis obliquus)	1
Removal of prosthetic medial collateral ligament	1
Miscellaneous	6
	21

In considering the use of synthetic ligaments for a prosthetic posterior cruciate ligament, there is noted to be a rather high incidence of subsequent procedures (Table 5). Most of these failures were related to the stresses placed on the ligament in the technique of insertion. It may well be that if this type of ligament is used at all in the future, the tapered ends should be removed, rounding out the ligament, and the ligament should be inserted in the center of the joint as suggested by Dr. KENNEDY. These modifications may obviate some of the mechanical disadvantages inherent in the original technique and improve the results.

In summary, perhaps by developing parameters of understanding in the entire scope of ligamentous instability of the knee, we can hope some day to develop realistic perspectives and incidentally delineate the potential role of prosthetic cruciate ligaments.

Discussion

JAKOB: I should like to add two observations concerning the isolated rupture of the anterior cruciate ligament and to the list of diagnostic features which you have given us. During the last two years, we have had three or four cases of confirmed isolated ruptures of the anterior cruciate ligament, and when these patients moved their knees actively or passively, they frequently complained of a pain in the back of the knee in the popliteal area which I cannot explain. I do not know if it has anything to do with the upper insertion or the origin of the anterior cruciate ligament which is partly extra-articular on the back side. Secondly, the only objective finding in absence of an anterior drawer sign has been just the beginning of a pivot syndrome. Therefore, if a patient with a history of such a "pop" event is being examined in case of effusion, we feel that if we do not find any anterior drawer sign or any medial laxity, we have to look very carefully for the pivot sign. In those cases which we were able to confirm afterwards by surgery, we were succesful with the sign. I would be interested in knowing what your experience has been.

BLAZINA: I would think that the pop or the pain posteriorly could be what you are describing as the more posterior position of the femoral insertion of the anterior cruciate ligament. There may be a hyperextension component to this, and you may have posterior capsular pain.

The criterion of no detectable instability which the West Point people used in diagnosis is confusing. I am not sure if it was made by clinical examination without anesthesia. They did not clarify that point. Perhaps if they had examined the patient under anesthesia there would have been some instability. Also, because of the position of the anterior cruciate ligament there was a mechanical block which may have forestalled the elucidation of some anterior instability or even a Pivot shift. I think that there is some play, but that was not what they described.

KARPF: Dr. BLAZINA'S lecture on the isolated tear of the anterior cruciate ligament was especially interesting for me because he said that primarily unstable knee joints become even more unstable and suffer cartilagenous damage after loss of the cruciate ligament. Will a joint which has only been stabilized medially and laterally become unstable again if the cruciate ligament is not also treated? Furthermore, do you operate the anterior cruciate ligament at all? How large must the drawer sign be before the indication for such an operation is given? Dr. KENNEDY said that with the drawer sign of over 10 mm the anterior cruciate ligament will also be operated. What methods would you use?

KENNEDY: I think those are good questions. As Dr. BLAZINA pointed out, we usually consider the anterior cruciate to be about 4 cm in overall length, if dissected from one end to the other. The middle two centimeters are the area where midcruciate tears commonly occur. Our experience has not been that satisfactory in acute primary repairs of this particular region. It is not that I disagree with repairs here; however, I think the outlook is not all that good as far as results are concerned. If, on the other hand, you do a meticulous repair in the upper third, the upper one centimeter, or directly at the bone, and providing you can place it far enough posteriorly and laterally, then your results are going to be reasonably good. As for patients who initially have a bit of a drawer sign but good collateral ligaments, we followed 50 of these over almost 8 years. During this period, the complications were slowly developing; at last check, 35% of that group were in some sort of trouble, but that still leaves 65% who were functioning pretty well with a known malfunction as far as the anterior cruciate was concerned. However, we tested many of these people with a clinical machine which tests the degree of instability in centimeters. It is possible to have a minor degree of anteroposterior damage where your two corners have gone posteromedial and posterolateral without any major varus or valgus instability. These patients seemed progressively to feel more pain when they trapped their medial or lateral meniscus or developed the so-called pivot shift or subluxation sign which we already discussed. For patients who get into a state where their anteroposterior instability is over 10 mm, we are now favoring the Eriksson operation. I just returned from Eriksson three days ago. He demonstrated an unselected group of 15 of his patients, and I got the impression that he and his colleagues do not see such badly unstable knees as we do in North America. Still, they had good results to show us.

WEBER: Dr. BLAZINA has told us that the West Point group had good results with about 30% of their cases in isolated anterior cruciate ligament sutures after 5 years. Have you an idea how the results would be without any operation at all?

BLAZINA: I think about the same.

JAMES: Dr. FEAGAN presented another follow-up this past March at one of the meetings at Sun Valley. I do not know in which he talked about this series and the follow-up on this particular group, but he entitled this talk "If I Knew Then What I Know Now." He explained his frustations with treating this type of injury; they were centered around the deterioration that you saw in this particular group of people.

BÖHLER: Dr. KENNEDY and Dr. JAMES, do you think it makes any sense at all to suture primarily an anterior cruciate ligament which is torn in the middle? Is not the vascularity then so bad that it has no chance to heal at all?

KENNEDY: That's my philosophy, but I still wouldn't discourage anyone from doing it. There's nothing to lose.

JAMES: I agree with Dr. KENNEDY. I am very pessimistic about a tear in that particular area.

JAKOB: Would you consider primary reconstuction in a midsubstance tear in an active sportsman?

KENNEDY: Some of our younger, enthusiastic orthopedic surgeons who look after a large volume of acute injuries are now doing immediate substitute operations for the acute midthird cruciate tears. Knowing what we do now, that philosophy may be a good one.

SCHULITZ: Dr. BLAZINA, do you have difficulties in finding the ligament when implanting the prosthetic ligament? The area of origin of the original ligament is relatively large; I would therefore like to ask which pole one should choose.

BLAZINA: I think that this was mentioned by me and by Dr. KENNEDY, at least in his previous talks. You must come in low on the tibia and you will usually place the hole a little more posteriorly than where

the anterior cruciate ligament ordinarily would come. If you bring it
too far forward you will have kinking of the ligament, and that may
lead to rupture. You cannot have a long ligament that will become kinked
or caught in extension. Therefore, the position of the anterior cruciate
ligament on the tibia is a little bit posterior to the ordinary insertion. The reverse situation happens with the posterior cruciate
ligament: it will come a little bit anterior to where the posterior
cruciate ligament usually inserts. Now of course for the anterior cruciate ligament on the femur, you should try to go back as far posteriorly as possible and make the femoral hole oblique so that you are almost
in a straight line. The femoral hole for the posterior cruciate ligament is very easy to do; it is just anterior to the articular cartilage.

BÖHLER: Dr. BLAZINA, you mentioned that up until a year ago you had no
method for an autogenous repair of the posterior cruciate. What do you
have now?

BLAZINA: Well, I think that the most popular operation in our country
within the last years has been the one utilizing the medial head of
the gastrocnemius. In my earlier discussion, I included a series of
figures on the Ellison and the modified Ellison procedure. I did this
because you will be reading literature in the next couple of years on
these procedures, and it will probably be advantageous for you to be
acquainted with this terminology. I also described certain other procedures relative to posterior instability. These are not my procedures
and are not procedures that I necessarily advocate. They have simply
been discussed by other people; you may hear about them, and, again,
I just wanted you to be familar with them. I would say the most popular
reconstruction of the posterior cruciate ligament in North America today is the medial head of the gastrocnemius.

BÖHLER: Could I pose the same question to the rest of the panel?

JAMES: I would give the same answer. We have been using the medial
head of the gastrocnemius for about five years. We were even using
that before the prosthetic ligament became available. Now it is being
used in conjunction with the prosthetic ligament in the hopes that
something will be there when the prosthetic ligament eventually ruptures, which the ones now available and in use are all going to do
eventually.

KENNEDY: I think my answer is about the same as that of Dr. JAMES.

O'DONOGHUE: I still use the semitendinosus, although I do not like it.

TRILLAT: I do not like to use the medial head of the gastrocnemius
because it seems to be very weak and very fine. Although it is difficult
to make a stable tendon inside the joint using the gracilis and the
semitendinosus, the combination of these two does create a ligament
which is relatively effective. On the other hand, one can use the gastrocnemius because it is well fixed when one has crossed the intercondylar space. It is easy to attach as well. It is stable, and experience proves that it is the best ligament for replacement.

MÜLLER: I would like to ask the surgeons who favor using the gastrocnemius whether they also fix it onto the tibia or whether they just
leave it on the tibia as it is. Do they just fasten the tendon above
onto the femur?

KENNEDY: In our situation I think that it is merely delivered from its
origin. It's high up, so you get all the tendon you can. We have actually tested its strength compared to that of other tendons around

the knee joint, and as we have found, it's by far the strongest tendon in that area. We make a small hole in the posterior capsule of the knee, deliver the tendon through, and then angle it forward in the femoral condyle. We do mobilize it a good deal down the tibia to gain the length we desire because often it is a bit short. The group in Houston, Texas, devised the little proplast ligament which Dr. BLAZINA had here. You can suture it to your medial head of the gastrocnemius while it is still in the popliteal fossa and then you bring it through. It gives you another 2 cm of length for tying; since it will become incorporated in the drill hole biologically, it does give you a little more play on your tendon.

MÜLLER: What do you do with that nerve branch entering the medial gastrocnemius head just above the joint level?

KENNEDY: I's about 1 cm distal to the muscular tendinous junction of the medial head, and it doesn't seem to be involved as you pull it through - which you must do with caution.

O'DONOGHUE: I can give the following tips for achieving adequate length with the semitendinosus transplant. You release it as far down the tibia as you can. You certainly have to pull the tendon tight. You then expose the back of the thighs and apply enough traction so that the muscles are in tension. After drilling a hole in the medial femoral condyle, you insert it into the condyle through the back of the joint, and then back to the tibia. It can be that you have trouble making the tibia hole oblique instead of coming through to the front; in this case it is just as well to come through the side to take what's left of the tendon. If you use this method. The semitendinosus is generally going to be long enough.

BLAZINA: One of the problems with autogenous ligamentous reconstructions has been fixation. However, as we continue our search for the perfected synthetic ligament which will involve the ultimate fixation, we will at the same time be able to improve fixation of tendinous transfers by the utilization of these materials, such as proplast or one of its prototypes with the capacity of fibrous tissue ingrowth. Eventually we will once again improve our autogenous reconstructions by utilizing techniques developed in the synthetic ligament research. This has already be done with methylmethycrylate using methylmethacrylate with wire sutures. It is like reinforced concrete and has been used in England with tendon transfers for paralytic disease. I think there will be a trading back and forth of knowledge in this field.

ROSSAK: Did you use lyophylized material?

BLAZINA: No.

MÜLLER: Do you make a second incision in the Lindemann procedure to fix the tibial head from behind?

TRILLAT: There are 3 surgeons including myself in our department who are concerned with this problem and who make different combined incisions. One surgeon only makes one large incision. The skin avulsions are very important. I personally prefer only one incision. In my opinion the smaller the cutaneous incision, the better the fixation.

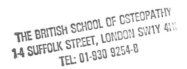

Subject Index

abduction stress test 77
adductor tubercle 80
anatomy of the knee 3
anterior cruciate ligament 5, 10, 12, 16, 17, 20, 23, 29, 34-36, 42, 76, 95, 106, 108, 114
anterior drawer sign 12, 17, 32, 35
anterior instability 110
anterolateral rotary instability 7, 9, 94, 110, 112
anteromedial retinaculum 82
anteromedial rotatory instability 5, 13, 86
anteroposterior instability 47
anteroposterior stability 43
arcuate ligament complex 7, 9, 35, 104
arcuate-popliteus-complex 34
arthrography, arthrogram 49, 52, 107
arthroscopy (arthroscopic examination) 49, 52, 55, 107
articular cartilage 53
assessment of chronic ligamentous instability 52

biceps muscle 9, 10
biceps tendon 34, 35, 65
bone-ligament preparation 20
bucket-handle tear 15

capsule 3
center of rotation 47
Check-List 52
chronic synovitis 29
classification of instability 33
cleavage leasions 54
collagen fibrils 21
combined instabilites 36
coronary ligaments 13
cruciate ligament 7, 9, 11, 44, 78
cuff of ligament 68
cyclic creep tests 24, 25

deep capsular ligament 4, 13

Ellison procedure 59, 60, 95
examination under anesthesia 56
extensor mechanism 51, 53

fatigue tests 24, 25
femoral condyle 7
femoral epicondyle 78
fibular collateral ligament 8, 9, 10, 34, 95, 103
foreign-body reaction 29

gastrocnemius 116
gastrocnemius insertion 6
gastrocnemius tendons, medial and lateral 7
geniculate artery 13
Gerdy's tubercle 9, 95
gracilis 116

Humphrey ligament 13, 15
hyperextension 12, 38
hyperextension valgus force 36

iliotibial band 95, 96
iliotibial tract 9, 11, 99
instability, anterior 110
    anterolateral 7, 110, 112
        rotatory 9, 94
    anteromedial 5, 13, 86
    anteroposterior 43, 47
    valgus 5
    varus 38
    posterolateral 7, 8, 99, 112, 112
    posteromedial 37
instant centers of rotation 38
Instron tension analyser 19
intraosseous fixation 28

jerk-test 84

knee anatomy 41
knee ligament instabilities 76

Lachman sign 18
lateral capsular ligament 35
lateral collateral ligament 7
lateral femoral condyle 12

lateral head of the gastrocnemius 9
lateral meniscus 7, 9, 15
lateral stability 9
lateral side injuries 43
Lenox Hill Brace 85
ligament of Humphrey 13, 15
ligamentous instability 53, 77
ligamentous reconstruction prodecures 58
loading forces 27
Location of injury 43
Losee test 94

mattres sutures 71
McIntosh repair 105
McIntosh test 9, 94
medial capsule 7, 80
medial capsular ligament 34, 36, 43
medial collateral ligament 39, 43, 70, 71, 74
medial instability of the knee 66
medial ligament instability 76
medial meniscectomy 59
medial meniscus 6, 7, 43, 80
medial posterior capsule 43
medial retinaculum 69
meniscal regeneration 54
meniscectomy 59, 78
menisci 13, 17, 53, 54, 78
method of examination 44
methyl-methacrylate cement 26
midlateral capsule 10

nerve supply 17
notch of the femur 9

oblique popliteal ligament 6, 7, 16
One-plane instabilities 34, 76

patellar stability 78
patellar tendon 78, 90, 109
patellar tendon transplant 83
pes anserinus 6, 69, 71, 78
pes anserinus transfer 83, 95
pes anserinus transplant 6, 76
Pivot-Shift-Test 9, 11, 94, 98, 114
Pivot-Syndrom 114
plastic module 30
Polyflex ligaments 22, 23
popliteal fascia 6
popliteus muscle 7, 9
popliteus tendon 7
posterior capsule 6-10, 34, 42, 43, 47, 71, 76, 80, 117
posterior cruciate ligament (posterior cruciate) 9, 12, 20, 29, 30, 34, 42, 43, 47, 70, 77, 103, 109, 111
posterior drawer sign 12

posterior horn of the medial meniscus 53
posterior instability 111
posterior oblique ligament complex 4, 16 17, 34-36, 76, 80, 81
posterolateral (and anterolateral) instability 7, 99, 104, 112
postero medial corner 70
posteromedial rotatory instability 37
prosthetic anterior cruciate ligaments 110, 112
prosthetic cruciate ligament 26, 27
prosthetic ligaments 92, 109 110, 116

rehabilative exercises 73
repeated hemarthrosis 31
residual elongation test 23
retinaculum 4
rotational instabilities 35, 76
rotatory instability test 77

saphenous nerve 7, 84, 90
sartorius muscle 80
sartorius, gracilis and semitendinosus muscles 6
scanning electron microscope 20
semimembranosus 70
semimembranosus tendon 4, 5, 7, 80, 81
semimembranosus transfer 64
semitendinosus 116
slocum maneuver 94
slocum test for rotatory instability 13, 77
stress X-ray 47, 49
surgical technique 68, 95
synovial biopsy 29
synthetic ligaments 113

tensile tests 24
tibia 81
tibial plateau 7
tibial tubercle 80
tibiocollateral ligament 4, 7, 20, 36, 76, 80
torsion tests 25

valgus and rotatory instability 5
valgus and varus instability 38, 115
vastus lateralis 9, 10
vastus medialis oblique muscle 7, 10
vascularization 31
visco-elastic properties 20

Wrisberg ligament 15

X-Ray 47, 49

Advances in Artificial Hip and Knee Joint Technology

Editors: M. Schaldach, D. Hohmann
In collaboration with R. Thull, F. Hein

1976. 525 figures. XII, 525 pages
(Engineering in Medicine, Volume 2)
Cloth DM 78,–; US $ 39.00
ISBN 3-540-07728-6

The Dynamic Compression Plate (DCP)

By M. Allgöwer, P. Matter, S. M. Perren, T. Rüedi

Revised Printing. 1978. 29 figures.
IV, 48 pages
DM 20,–; US $ 10.00
ISBN 3-540-06466-4

H.-R. Henche

Die Arthroskopie des Kniegelenks

Mit einem Geleitwort von E. Morscher

1978. 163 Abbildungen, davon 66 farbig,
1 Tabelle. X, 86 Seiten
Gebunden DM 128,–; US $ 64.00
ISBN 3-540-08380-4

R. Liechti

Hip Arthrodesis and Its Problems

Foreword by M. E. Müller, B. G. Weber
Translated from the German edition "Die
Arthrodese des Hüftgelenkes und ihre
Problematik" by P. A. Casey

1978. 266 figures, 7 tables.
Approx. 280 pages
Cloth DM 128,–; US $ 64.00
ISBN 3-540-08614-5

Die Frakturenbehandlung bei Kindern und Jugendlichen

Herausgeber: B. G. Weber, C. Brunner,
F. Freuler
Unter Mitarbeit zahlreicher Fach-
wissenschaftler

1978. 462 Abbildungen, 27 Tabellen.
X, 414 Seiten
Gebunden DM 278,–; US $ 139.00
ISBN 3-540-08299-9

P. G. J. Maquet

Biomechanics of the Knee

With Application to the Pathogenesis and
the Surgical Treatment of Osteoarthritis

1976. 184 figures. XIII, 230 pages
Cloth DM 168,–; US $ 84.00
ISBN 3-540-07882-7

Prices are subject to change without notice

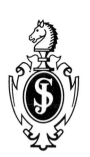

Springer-Verlag
Berlin
Heidelberg
New York

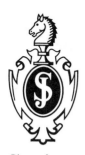